KETOGENIC DIET AND RECIPES

WHY YOU SHOULD TRY IT

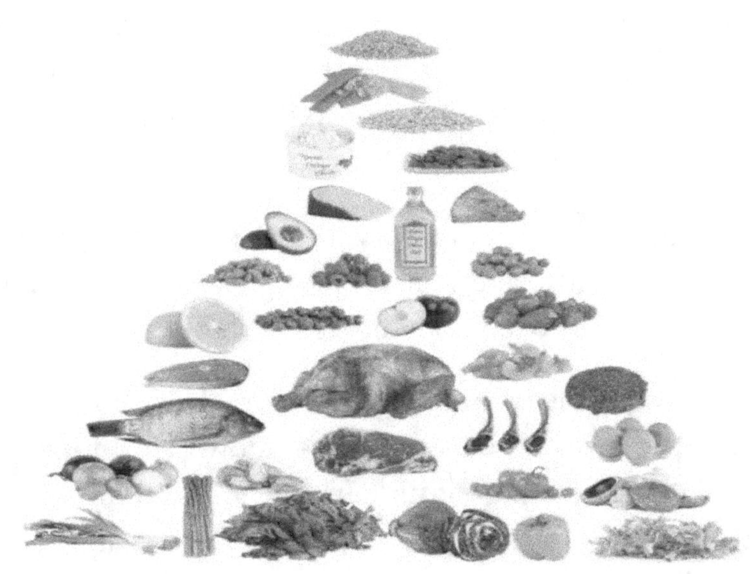

BY BEVERLY HILL

Introduction

I want to thank you and congratulate you for choosing the book, *"**KETOGENIC DIET AND RECIPES: WHY YOU SHOULD TRY IT** "*.

The ketogenic diet, aka the "keto diet," is low in carbohydrates and high in good fats, and it provides you with a lot of energy. The idea of this type of diet is by eating foods that are high in fats, it will provide you with a numerous amount of energy. The idea is that by eating high-fat foods, moderate-protein, and fewer carbs., the body goes into ketosis, or the metabolic state in which ketone bodies (fat-like molecules) become the main fuel source instead of glucose.

Ketogenic diets is said to be very effective at diabetes control, lowering blood glucose levels, and reducing weight when you eat about 30 grams of carbohydrates per day or below.

This encourages the body to get its energy from burning body fat which produces an energy source known as ketones. The diet helps to lower the body's demand for insulin which has benefits for people with type 1 and type 2 diabetes. People on insulin will typically require smaller doses of insulin which leads to less risk of large dosing errors. The diet helps burn body fat, and therefore has advantages for those looking to lose weight, including people with prediabetes, or those otherwise at risk of type 2 diabetes.

How do you add "keto diet" into your daily routine? When meal planning, you're aiming to get 70 to 75 percent of your calories from fat, 20 to 25 percent from protein, and 5 to 10 percent from carbohydrates. You're allowed to eat whole, unprocessed foods ones that are high in fat and protein, along with a few complex carbs. High-carb foods are completely cut out so say goodbye to grains, potatoes, beans, syrups, pastries, fruit, and even milk. Basically, if it tastes sweet or has an "-ose" on the end, you're going to have to ditch it. Why? Because studies have found endurance athletes who eat low-carb and high-fat burn more fat during their performances compared to their carb-eating peers.

It all sounds pretty good, right? Before you drop everything, here are a few more things you should know. The keto diet was not orginally intended for weight loss or to help athletes perform better. Instead, it was created in the early 20th century to help children with epilepsy control their seizures.

Before the keto diet was introduced most epileptic patients were advised to fast, but that proved to be difficult for many. It was found that eating high-fat and low-carb, it produced the same metabolic changes as the fasting approach, which meant increased liver production of three molecules (keton bodies) acetone, 3-hydroxydutyrate, and acetoacetate. It's still unclear to experts why it helps, but for now, it's working.

Thanks again for choosing this book, I hope you enjoy it!

ABOUT THE AUTHOR

Beverly Hill is a sociologist. She is the CEO of C.E.F Associates and formerly served as head of department of sociology in Premier Natural Resources Inc.

A graduate of Nelson High School also graduated from the University of Toronto with a B.A in economics and finance and holds an M.S from Cambridge University in public relations and PhD in sociology.

She has written many articles on human equality, animal rights, environmental issues, personal development and peace keeping in different newspapers. She has also appeared in many magazines and is frequently interviewed for articles on family, race, socioeconomic status, and how to survive in your environment. She has also worked on the importance of health of relationship between parents and children. Her book 'The Middle Child' focuses on the importance of the attention given to the children and what to expect from them. This book helps parents understand their children.

In addition to these works she is also the author of 'Surviving Alone ' which is about her own childhood growing up; she writes about her family struggles living on a low income budget and growing her own food to survive.

C.E.F Associates formed in 1999 in Idaho, USA she worked both nationally and internationally. This is a consulting company which has clients all over the world. Ms. Hill the CEO of the company is the main reason of the huge client base because of her servings in foreign countries.

TABLE OF CONTENT

Chapter 1

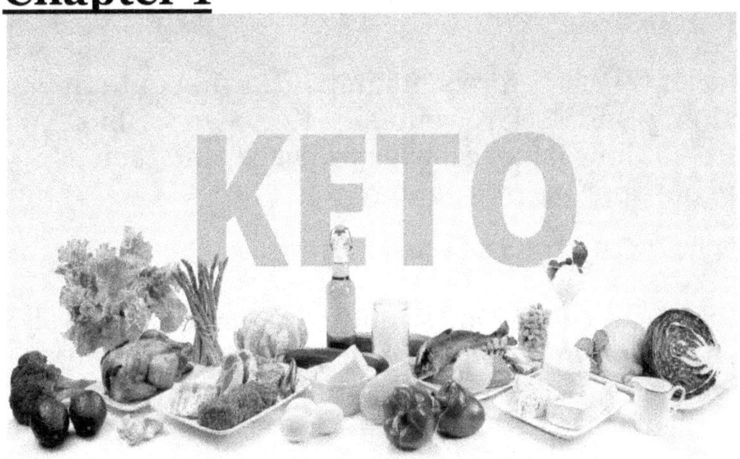

HOW TO START THE KETO DIET

You've seen the research. You've read the stories of people improving their health, losing weight, and feeling mentally sharp. Now, you've decided it's your turn to reap the benefits of keto, too. But what if you're stuck on exactly HOW to start ketogenic diet the right way? No worries, the hardest part is starting, right? You've already made the first step, so let's help you begin in style.

First, know that a huge part of succeeding on the keto diet is all about the food and correct ratios. You're literally using the macronutrients of what you eat to change your body chemistry.

Let's have a brief, basic lesson on metabolism:

Under normal circumstances, the body burns carbohydrates as its primary source of fuel. When you start eating a ketogenic diet, you "starve" your body of those carbohydrate sources by eating very low carb.

When no carbs are present for the body to utilize, it will start breaking down fat for fuel, and start producing what are known as ketone bodies, or ketones, for energy. By doing this, you're teaching your body to start burning FAT for fuel instead of carbs because you're greatly reducing the amount of carbs you giving your body.

Pretty great, right? But before you jump head-first onto the low-carb training, and declare yourself a Ketonian for life. You need to figure out how many calories you need, and then use that to figure out your macros per day.

PROTEIN ON THE KETOGENIC DIET

It's important to carefully monitor not only your ketone levels, but also your amount of protein. While protein is certainly important for health, it's also a tricky subject when you're on the ketogenic diet.

In the presence of carbohydrates, the body will either turn to protein or fat for fuel, and if your protein is too high, it'll start to break it down instead. This is known as gluconeogenesis, which is a process that converts excess protein into glycogen to keep your body burning glucose as its primary fuel. Which means your lean muscle mass will fall victim to your body, and that's bad news. You want to keep your muscle so you don't waste away.

But it's okay because, as I've discussed above, keto involves keeping your protein count moderate, not high, so you can keep on burning that extra fat while also keeping your healthy muscle tone.

MEASURING YOUR KETONE LEVELS

Besides being strict with your macro ratios, the other half of success on a ketogenic diet is tracking. You MUST consistently track your ketone levels to really know how the keto diet is working for you, and to notice any areas that need tweaking.

There are three main ways to test your ketone levels:

1. Blood testing

2. Urine testing

3. Breath testing

Each method has its place, but blood testing is where it's at if you want an accurate view of your ketosis level.

FASTING TO GET INTO KETOSIS FASTER

One method some keto dieters use to get into ketosis quickly is by fasting.

You can get into ketosis without fasting, of course, but you might find it happening much faster with fasting, so it's something to consider.

Exogenous ketones are another great resource for kicking yourself into ketosis sooner, and having plenty of ketone bodies available for energy.

If you're ready to start a ketogenic diet today, this will get you started. Get to know your favorite whole food, high-fat, and especially animal-based sources of fat and protein, invest in a blood meter for testing those ketones, stock up on some extra ketones for the ride, and get ready to make a significant change for your body and your health!

The two other types of the diet haven't been fully tested yet. However, there are some stated benefits.

When you want to add some carbs to a workout, you can follow the targeted ketogenic diet. You're allowed a few extra carbs, but they are only on the days and the time of your workouts. The focus is on getting the exercise without struggling with energy. You wouldn't need to do this if you get enough fat into your diet, and once your body gets into the ketone producing zone.

The cyclical diet is another one that focuses on more carbs. This is more of a cycle hence the name. You'll get five days where you follow the standard diet, and then two days where you get more carbs. This sort of diet could be perfect for those who struggle to stick to a plan or just know they wouldn't be able to last without any potatoes, bread or pasta at all. Think of this like your 5:2 diet, where you get two days off.

Now it's your turn. Pick your diet and choose from the best keto recipes for weight loss share below.

GETTING STARTED

Getting started on the keto diet can sound like hard work. There's so much to learn, and so much to remember: What to eat, what to avoid, and how to take those critical first steps when you begin.

Below, I've put together a list of things you should know before you start the keto diet by making sure you're prepared, and give you the best possible chance of success. It's important to clear up any misconceptions before you begin to make sure you start the keto diet the healthy way. And luckily, getting started isn't as complicated as you might think.

BENEFITS OF THE KETO DIET

1. LOSE WEIGHT

It's not clear why the ketogenic diet is so great for weight loss, but as this review states, "there is no doubt that there is strong supportive evidence that the use of ketogenic diets in weight loss therapy is effective."

2. CURB YOUR CRAVINGS

By balancing your blood sugar levels. Many of our cravings are caused by swings in our blood sugar (due to eating carbohydrates and sugary foods) so eliminating carbs gets rid of this problem.

3. CURB HUNGER AND REDUCE OVEREATING

It's unclear whether ketosis, high fat, high protein, or low carb creates this effect, but studies have shown that a ketogenic diet (especially one high in protein) can curb your appetite naturally.

4. INCREASE YOUR FOCUS

Also, it help you be more alert and focused. Your mind will be clearer and sharper, and you'll no longer suffer from the dreaded "mid-afternoon slump" that has so many people reaching for cookies and more coffee.

5. ALZHEIMER'S, CANCER, AND CARDIOVASCULAR DISEASE

There is a 'hidden face' of the ketogenic diet: Its broader therapeutic action. And its potential in aiding the treatment and prevention of cancer, cardiovascular, and neurological diseases are some of the most exciting possibilities.

THINGS TO KNOW ABOUT THE KETO DIET BEFORE YOU GET STARTED

1. Food quality still matters which means eating high-quality nutrient dense foods, and avoiding processed junk foods (even if they're low carb).

2. Keto is more than just eating low carb so adding more healthy fats to your diet is vital. But if you're not used to eating so much fat, increase your fat intake gradually – otherwise it can give you digestive issues.

3. Higher ketone levels aren't essential for weight loss, and the ketone level you want to achieve can vary depending on a few factors.

4. Measuring your ketone levels isn't compulsory, but it can be a good way to ensure you've reached nutritional ketosis, and to troubleshoot any problems.

5. What you eat isn't everything ...it's also important to get enough sleep, manage your stress levels, and make time to exercise. A keto diet should be just one part of an overall healthy lifestyle: That is, if you're not taking care of yourself, a keto diet won't fix things.

6. Keto can be tough in the beginning while your body adapts to burning fat instead of glucose. Be prepared for this, and make sure you have a powerful reason for starting keto to keep you motivated while you get through it. If you find you're suffering from uncomfortable symptoms (also called keto flu).

7. Getting health tests before you start can be a good idea, to make sure any underlying issues like autoimmune conditions, gut problems, and vitamin/mineral deficiencies are taken care of. This allows you to get the full benefits of the keto diet when you try it.

HOW DO YOU GET STARTED ON KETO?

Clear out your kitchen and get rid of all your non-keto food, especially any sweet treats you have lying around. It's easier to stick to your diet if there's nothing to tempt you!

Start your day with a ketone boosting ritual by drinking a large glass of water, and taking two teaspoons of coconut oil, or half a teaspoon of MCT oil.

Choose one meal each day to skip as it makes eating keto a lot easier if you only have to think about two meals each day.

Why not try skipping dinner, and going to bed early as well this will also help reset your circadian rhythm!

Eat unlimited protein/fat in the beginning, but stick to under 25g of carbohydrates per day.

Its best to keep things simple when you begin, and alter your protein/fat ratios later, when you're more used to the keto way of eating.

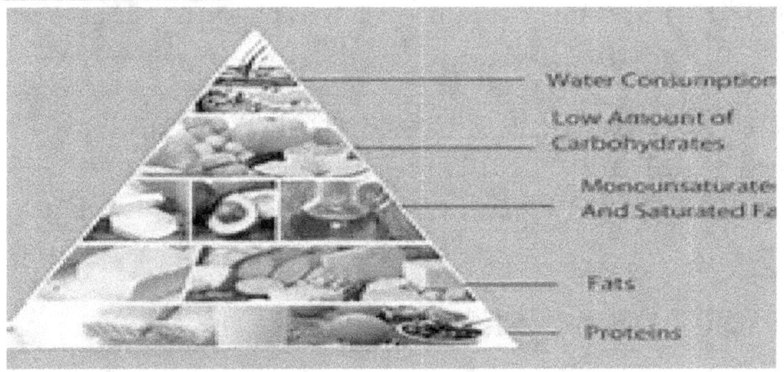

Chapter 2

A DETAILED BEGINNER'S GUIDE

The ketogenic diet is a low-carb, high-fat diet that offers many health benefits.

Studies show that this type of diet can help you lose weight, and improve health.

Ketogenic diets may even have benefits against diabetes, cancer, epilepsy, and Alzheimer's disease.

What is a Ketogenic Diet?

The ketogenic diet (often termed keto) is a very low-carb, high-fat diet that shares many similarities with the Atkins and low-carb diets.

It involves drastically reducing carbohydrate intake, and replacing it with fat. The reduction in carbs puts your body into a metabolic state called ketosis.

When this happens, your body becomes incredibly efficient at burning fat for energy. It also turns fat into ketones in the liver, which can supply energy for the brain.

Ketogenic diets can cause massive reductions in blood sugar and insulin levels. This, along with the increased ketones, has numerous health benefits.

The ketogenic diet (keto) is a low-carb, high-fat diet. It lowers blood sugar and insulin levels, and shifts the body's metabolism away from carbs and towards fat and ketones.

Different Types of Ketogenic Diets

There are several versions of the ketogenic diet, including:

Standard ketogenic diet (SKD): This is a very low-carb, moderate-protein and high-fat diet. It typically contain 75% fat, 20% protein and only 5% carbs.

Cyclical ketogenic diet (CKD): This diet involves periods of higher-carb refeeds, such as 5 ketogenic days followed by 2 high-carb days.

Targeted ketogenic diet (TKD): This diet allows you to add carbs around workouts.

High-protein ketogenic diet: This is similar to a standard ketogenic diet, but includes more protein. The ratio is often 60% fat, 35% protein and 5% carbs.

However, only the standard and high-protein ketogenic diets have been studied extensively. Cyclical or targeted ketogenic diets are more advanced methods, and primarily used by bodybuilders or athletes.

Although there are several versions of the ketogenic diet. The standard ketogenic diet (SKD) is the most researched and most recommended.

Ketogenic Diets Can Help You Lose Weight

A ketogenic diet is an effective way to lose weight and lower risk factors for disease.

In fact, research shows that the ketogenic diet is far superior to the recommended low-fat diet. The diet is so filling that you can lose weight without counting calories or tracking your food.

One study found that people on a ketogenic diet lost 2.2 times more weight than those on a calorie-restricted low-fat diet. Triglyceride and HDL cholesterol levels also improved.

Another study found that participants on the ketogenic diet lost 3 times more weight than those on the Diabetes UK's recommended diet.

There are several reasons why a ketogenic diet is superior to a low-fat diet. One is the increased protein intake, which provides numerous benefits.

The increased ketones, lowered blood sugar levels and improved insulin sensitivity may also play a key role.

A ketogenic diet can help you lose much more weight than a low-fat diet. This often happens without hunger.

Ketogenic Diets for Diabetes and Prediabetes

Diabetes is characterized by the changes in metabolism, high blood sugar and impaired insulin function.

The ketogenic diet can help you lose excess fat, which is closely linked to type 2 diabetes, prediabetes and metabolic syndrome.

One study found that the ketogenic diet improved insulin sensitivity by a whopping 75%.

Another study in patients with type 2 diabetes found that 7 of the 21 participants were able to stop all diabetes medications.

In another study, the ketogenic group lost 24.4 lbs (11.1 kg), compared to 15.2 lbs (6.9 kg) in the higher-carb group. This is an important benefit when considering the link between weight and type 2 diabetes.

Additionally, 95.2% of the ketogenic group is also able to stop or reduce diabetes medication, compared to 62% in the higher-carb group.

The ketogenic diet can boost insulin sensitivity and cause fat loss, leading to drastic improvement for type 2 diabetes and prediabetes.

Other Health Benefits of the Ketogenic Diet

The ketogenic diet actually originated as a tool for treating neurological diseases, such as epilepsy.

Studies have shown that the diet can have benefits for a wide variety of different health conditions such as:

Heart disease: The ketogenic diet can improve risk factors like body fat, HDL levels, blood pressure and blood sugar.

Cancer: The diet is currently being used to treat several types of cancer and slow tumor growth.

Alzheimer's disease: The diet may reduce symptoms of Alzheimer's, and slow down the disease's progression.

Epilepsy: Research has shown that the ketogenic diet can cause massive reductions in seizures in epileptic children.

Parkinson's disease: One study found that the diet helped improve symptoms of Parkinson's disease.

Polycystic ovary syndrome: The ketogenic diet can help reduce insulin levels, which may play a key role in polycystic ovary syndrome.

Brain injuries: One animal study found that the diet can reduce concussions, and aid recovery after brain injury.

Acne: Lower insulin levels and eating less sugar or processed foods may help improve acne.

However, keep in mind that research into many of these areas is far from conclusive.

A ketogenic diet may provide many health benefits, especially with metabolic, neurological or insulin-related diseases.

FOODS TO AVOID

In short, any food that is high in carbs should be limited.

Here is a list of foods that need to be reduced or eliminated on a ketogenic diet:

Sugary foods: Soda, fruit juice, smoothies, cake, ice cream, candy, etc.

Grains or starches: Wheat-based products, rice, pasta, cereal, etc.

Fruit: All fruit, except small portions of berries like strawberries.

Beans or legumes: Peas, kidney beans, lentils, chickpeas, etc.

Root vegetables and tubers: Potatoes, sweet potatoes, carrots, parsnips, etc.

Low-fat or diet products: These are highly processed and often high in carbs.

Some condiments or sauces: These often contain sugar and unhealthy fat.

Unhealthy fat: Limit your intake of processed vegetable oils, mayonnaise, etc.

Alcohol: Due to its carb content, many alcoholic beverages can throw you out of ketosis.

Sugar-free diet foods: These are often high in sugar alcohols, which can affect ketone levels in some cases. These foods also tend to be highly processed.

Avoid carb-based foods like grains, sugars, legumes, rice, potatoes, candy, juice and even most fruits.

FOODS TO EAT

You should base the majority of your meals around these foods:

Meat: Red meat, steak, ham, sausage, bacon, chicken and turkey.

Fatty fish: Such as, salmon, trout, tuna and mackerel.

Eggs: Look for pastured or omega-3 whole eggs.

Butter and cream: Look for grass-fed when possible.

Cheese: Unprocessed cheese (cheddar, goat, cream, blue or mozzarella).

Nuts and seeds: Almonds, walnuts, flaxseeds, pumpkin seeds, chia seeds, etc.

Healthy oils: Primarily extra virgin olive oil, coconut oil, and avocado oil.

Avocados: Whole avocados or freshly made guacamole.

Low-carb veggies: Most green veggies, tomatoes, onions, peppers, etc.

Condiments: You can use salt, pepper and various healthy herbs and spices.

Base the majority of your diet on foods such as meat, fish, eggs, butter, nuts, healthy oils, avocados, and plenty of low-carb veggies.

KETOGENIC MEAL PLAN FOR 1 WEEK

To help get you started, here is a sample ketogenic diet meal plan for one week:

Monday

Breakfast: Bacon, eggs and tomatoes.

Lunch: Chicken salad with olive oil and feta cheese.

Dinner: Salmon with asparagus cooked in butter.

Tuesday

Breakfast: Egg, tomato, basil and goat cheese omelet.

Lunch: Almond milk, peanut butter, cocoa powder and stevia milkshake.

Dinner: Meatballs, cheddar cheese and vegetables.

Wednesday

Breakfast: A ketogenic milkshake.

Lunch: Shrimp salad with olive oil and avocado.

Dinner: Pork chops with Parmesan cheese, broccoli and salad.

Thursday

Breakfast: Omelet with avocado, salsa, peppers, onion and spices.

Lunch: A handful of nuts, and celery sticks with guacamole and salsa.

Dinner: Chicken stuffed with pesto and cream cheese, along with vegetables.

Friday

Breakfast: Sugar-free yogurt with peanut butter, cocoa powder, and stevia.

Lunch: Beef stir-fry cooked in coconut oil with vegetables.

Dinner: Bun-less burger with bacon, egg and cheese.

Saturday

Breakfast: Ham and cheese omelet with vegetables.

Lunch: Ham and cheese slices with nuts.

Dinner: White fish, egg and spinach cooked in coconut oil.

Sunday

Breakfast: Fried eggs with bacon and mushrooms.

Lunch: Burger with salsa, cheese and guacamole.

Dinner: Steak and eggs with a side salad.

Always try to rotate the vegetables and meat over the long term, as each type provides different nutrients and health benefits.

You can eat a wide variety of tasty and nutritious meals on a ketogenic diet.

Healthy Ketogenic Snacks

Here is a list of healthy ketogenic snacks:

Fatty meat or fish.

Cheese.

A handful of nuts or seeds.

Cheese with olives.

1–2 hard-boiled eggs.

90% dark chocolate.

A low-carb milk shake with almond milk, cocoa powder and nut butter.

Full-fat yogurt mixed with nut butter and cocoa powder.

Strawberries and cream.

Celery with salsa and guacamole.

Smaller portions of leftover meals.

Great snacks for a keto diet include pieces of meat, cheese, olives, boiled eggs, nuts, and dark chocolate.

Tips for Eating Out on a Ketogenic Diet

It's not very hard to make most restaurant meals keto-friendly when eating out.

Most restaurants offer some meat or fish-based dishes. Order this, and replace any high-carb food with extra vegetables.

Egg-based meals are also a great option, such as an omelet or eggs and bacon.

Another favorite is bun-less burgers. You could also leave the bun and swap the fries for vegetables instead. Add extra avocado, cheese, bacon or eggs.

For dessert, ask for a mixed cheese board or double cream with berries.

When eating out, select a meat, fish or egg-based dish. Order extra veggies instead of carbs or starches, and have cheese for dessert.

Side Effects and How to Minimize Them

Although the ketogenic diet is safe for healthy people, there may be some initial side effects while your body adapts.

This is often referred to as "keto flu" - and is usually over within a few days.

Keto flu includes poor energy and mental function, increased hunger, sleep issues, nausea, digestive discomfort, and decreased exercise performance.

In order to minimize this, you can try a regular low-carb diet for the first few weeks. This teaches your body to burn more fat before you completely eliminate carbs.

A ketogenic diet can also change the water and mineral balance of your body, so adding extra salt to your meals or taking mineral supplements can help.

For minerals, try taking 3,000–4,000 mg of sodium, 1,000 mg of potassium, and 300 mg of magnesium per day to minimize side effects.

At least in the beginning, it is important to eat until fullness, and to avoid restricting calories too much. Usually a ketogenic diet causes weight loss without intentional calorie restriction.

Many of the side effects of starting a ketogenic diet can be limited. Easing into the diet, and taking mineral supplements can help.

Supplements For a Ketogenic Diet

Although no supplement is necessary, some can be useful.

Medium-Chain Triglycerides (MCT) oil: Added to drinks or yogurt, MCT oil provides energy, and helps increase ketone levels.

Minerals: Added salt and other minerals can be important when starting out, due to shifts in water and mineral balance.

Caffeine: Caffeine can have benefits for energy, fat loss and performance.

Exogenous ketones: This supplement can help raise the body's ketone levels.

Creatine: Creatine provides numerous benefits for health and performance. This can help if you are combining a ketogenic diet with exercise.

Whey: Use half a scoop of whey protein in shakes or yogurt to increase your daily protein intake.

Certain supplements can be beneficial on a ketogenic diet. These include exogenous ketones, MCT oil, and minerals.

FREQUENTLY ASKED QUESTIONS

1. Can I ever eat carbs again?

Yes. However, it is important to eliminate them initially. After the first 2–3 months, you can eat carbs on special occasions; just return to the diet immediately after.

2. Will I lose muscle?

There is a risk of losing some muscle on any diet. However, the high protein intake, and high ketone levels may help minimize muscle loss, especially if you lift weights.

3. Can you build muscle on a ketogenic diet?

Yes, but it may not work as well as on a moderate-carb diet. More details can be found if you search: Low-Carb/Ketogenic Diets, and Exercise Performance.

4. Do I need to refeed or carb load?

No. However, a few higher-calorie days may be beneficial every now and then.

5. How much protein can I eat?

Protein should be moderate, as a very high intake can spike insulin levels and lower ketones. Around 35% of total calorie intake is probably the upper limit.

6. What if I am constantly tired, weak or fatigued?

You may not be in full ketosis or be utilizing fats and ketones efficiently. To counter this, lower your carb intake, and re-visit the points above. A supplement like MCT oil or ketones may also help.

7. My urine smells fruity? Why is this?

Don't be alarmed. This is simply due to the excretion of byproducts created during ketosis.

8. My breath smells. What can I do?

This is a common side effect. Try drinking naturally flavored water or chewing sugar-free gum.

9. I heard ketosis was extremely dangerous. Is this true?

People often confuse ketosis with ketoacidosis. The former is natural, while the latter only occurs in uncontrolled diabetes.

Ketoacidosis is dangerous, but the ketosis on a ketogenic diet is perfectly normal and healthy.

10. I have digestion issues and diarrhea. What can I do?

This common side effect usually passes after 3–4 weeks. If it persists, try eating more high-fiber veggies. Magnesium supplements can also help with constipation.

A Ketogenic Diet is Great, But Not For Everyone

A ketogenic diet can be great for people who are overweight, diabetic or looking to improve their metabolic health. It may be less suitable for elite athletes or those wishing to add large amounts of muscle or weight.

And, as with any diet, it will only work if you are consistent, and stick with it in the long-term.

That being said, few things are as well proven in nutrition as the powerful health and weight loss benefits of a ketogenic diet. Please consult with your doctor before trying any diet.

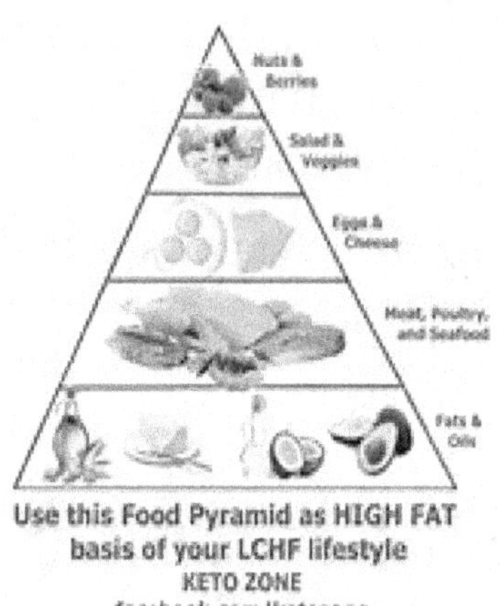

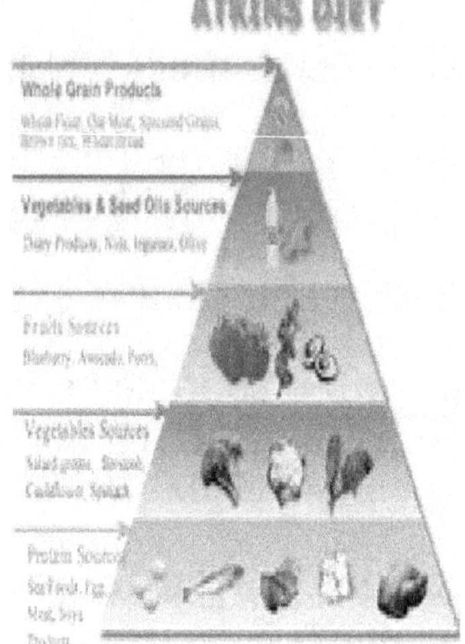

Chapter 3

WHAT IS A KETOGENIC DIET, AND HOW DOES IT RELATE TO THE AKINS DIET

You've probably heard plenty about the Atkins Diet over the years. You know, that incredibly popular and controversial diet that involves cutting right down on your carbohydrate intake. You may also heard of "ketogenic diets" - it's a more scientific term so you may not recognise it. Did you realise that the Atkins Diet is a type of ketogenic diet?   I'll have a brief look at what the term means, and my experience of this type of diet.

The Atkins Diet

Dr. Atkins' Diet Revolution, was released in 1972. Dr Robert Atkins was interested, among other things, in getting his own weight under control. Primarily using self-experimentation techniques he found that eating a diet very low in carbohydrates tended to make him lose weight quickly.

His experimentation was based upon other research papers, and as a result of his own studies, he became confident that the science behind the diet was sound. The resulting book was a resounding success, and over the next 30 years up to his death in 2003, Robert Atkins continued to produce popular diet books based upon the low-carbohydrate principle.

Ketogenic Diets

Some would argue that the first "phase" of the Atkins Diet is "ketogenic", but it's very clear that this element is central to the whole diet. There are many other diets of this type with different names and claims, but if they talk about severely restricting the intake of carbohydrates, then they're probably forms of ketogenic diet. The process of "ketosis" is quite complicated, and would take some time to describe, but in essence, it works because cutting down on carbs restricts the amount of blood glucose available to trigger the "insulin response."

Without a triggering of the glucose-insulin response some hormonal changes take place which cause the body to start burning its stores of fat as energy. This also has the interesting effect of causing your brain to be fuelled by what are known as "ketone bodies" (hence "ketogenic") rather than the usual glucose. The whole process is really fascinating, and I recommend that you read up on it.

 All forms of ketogenic diet are controversial. Most of the debate surrounds the issue of cholesterol, and whether ketogenic diets increase or decrease the levels HDL or "good" cholesterol and/or increase or decrease LDL or "bad" cholesterol. ,The number of scientific studies is increasing year on year and it is certainly possible to point to strong cases on both sides of the argument.

One could equally make the case that a carbohydrate-laden diet has negative effects on cholesterol, and I think that on balance, a ketogenic-type diet is more healthy than a carbohydrate-heavy one. Interestingly, there isn't so much controversy about whether ketogenic diets work or not (it's widely accepted that they do); it's about how they work, and whether that is good/bad/or indifferent from a health perspective.

It's difficult, if you are just starting out looking for a diet that works for you, to know where the truth lies in this debate; if the scientists can't sort it out then how are you going to? The truth is that you'll need to educate yourself, weigh the arguments, then follow your own best judgement. Research has been largely positive, but you will no doubt, have heard of friends having problems on low carbohydrate diets for one reason or another.

There is no such thing as a miracle diet, and most of them are just variations on a theme, but all ketogenic-type diets are based upon a very specific principle, and that principle has been demonstrated to induce weight loss in many people. Perhaps you should try to base your opinion on the available evidence, and not on anecdotes. After all, it's your body and your health.

Chapter 4

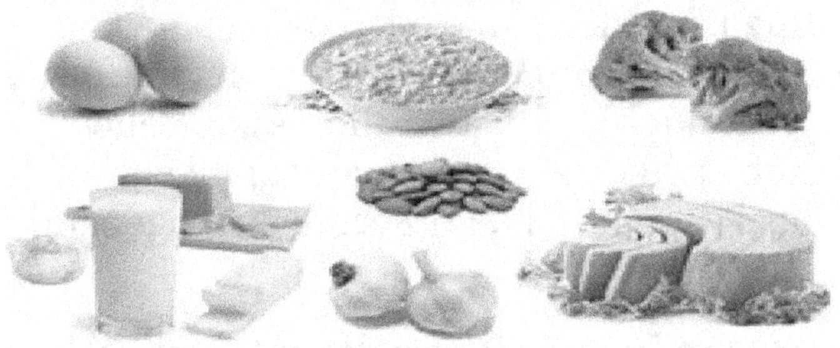

THE BEST FAT BURNING DIET

For the best diet to rapidly burn fat using the body's natural metabolism, consider a ketogenic diet plan. Nutrition has the strongest effect on the body's production of important hormones, which regulate metabolism, and allow the body to burn fat for energy, and retain muscle mass, with little need for excessive exercise.

What is a ketogenic diet plan?

Basically, it is a diet that causes the body to enter a state of ketosis. Ketosis is a natural and healthy metabolic state in which the body burns its own stored fat (producing ketones), instead of using glucose (the sugars from carbohydrates found in the Standard American Diet - SAD).

Metabolically speaking, ketogenic foods are very powerful. The amazing benefit is these foods are also delicious, natural whole foods that are extremely healthy for you.

So what foods are encouraged?

Some of the best-tasting, most fulfilling foods are part of this plan, including lean meats like beef and chicken, healthy sources of protein, and high-quality fats like eggs, butter, olive oil, coconut oil, and avocado. Also, delicious leafy-green vegetables like kale, chard, and spinach, as well as cruciferous vegetables like broccoli, cabbage, and cauliflower.

These foods can be combined with seeds, nuts, sprouts, and a wide range of other amazing foods that lead to incredible health benefits that give your body the protein, healthy fats, and nutrients it needs while providing metabolism-boosting meals for easy cooking at home or on the go.

What foods should be limited?

On a ketogenic diet plan, the main foods to avoid are those high in carbohydrates, sugars, and the wrong types of fats. These foods can be toxic to the body, and create excess glucose levels that the body turns into stored fat. Also, they can increase the level of insulin and blood sugar in the body, and will prevent fat loss even if you are putting a lot of energy into exercise. To avoid these foods, limit your intake of grains, processed foods, vegetable oils (canola, corn, soybean, etc.), milk, margarine, and other high-carbohydrate, high-sugar foods.

But, aren't fats bad for you?

We have been told for decades that calories from fats should be reduced to encourage weight loss, but this is a vast over-simplification (still supported by government and industrial food interests) that is no longer accurate according our modern understanding of human nutrition. The reality is that certain fats are not good for you (those high in omega-6 fatty acids), because your body has a hard time processing them. Other fats, particularly medium chain triglycerides (MCTs), are extremely beneficial for weight loss, brain cell generation, and nutrients. These healthy saturated fats should be increased to give your body the energy it needs while in ketosis, while limiting the detrimental trans-fats found in many processed foods.

What are the benefits of a ketogenic diet plan?

1. **Burn Stored Fat** - By cutting out the high levels of carbohydrates in your diet that produce glucose (sugar), a ketogenic diet plan tells your body to burn stored fat by converting this fat into fatty acids and ketone bodies in the liver. These ketone bodies replace the role of glucose that was being filled by carbohydrates in the diet. This leads to a rapid reduction in the amount of fat stored in the body.

2. **Retain Muscle Mass** - By including the right fats in your diet, a ketogenic diet plan provides your body with the energy it needs to convert existing fat stores into useful sugars and ketones (through gluconeogenesis), which are an essential source of energy for the brain, muscles, and heart. This has the added benefit of preserving muscle mass, because the healthy fat in the diet gives the body the energy it needs without having to tap into muscle protein to create more sugar. This creates the best of both worlds - burn fat while maintaining muscle mass!

3. **Eliminate Excess Fat** - If your body creates too many ketone bodies by converting existing fat, it

will simply eliminate those ketones as a waste product.

4. **Reduce Appetite** - Lastly, by regulating the powerful metabolic hormones in your body, a ketogenic diet plan will actually reduce your appetite. By lowering your body's insulin resistance and increasing ketones, you will actually feel less hungry on this diet, which is an amazing advantage over other low-calorie, carbohydrate-rich weight loss diets that come with the expectation of lingering hunger.

Start burning fat today without more exercise! Take control of your metabolism naturally by adopting a ketogenic diet plan. Your body was designed for this style of nutrition. Your metabolic state can be optimized by consuming the (delicious) foods that our genetic forefathers thrived on, and this does not include carbohydrate-rich, processed foods loaded with sugars, and bad fats. It involves a luxurious and fulfilling diet based on bountiful foods from paleolithic times, including lean meats, vegetables, nuts and seeds, and healthy fats that your body will thank you for.

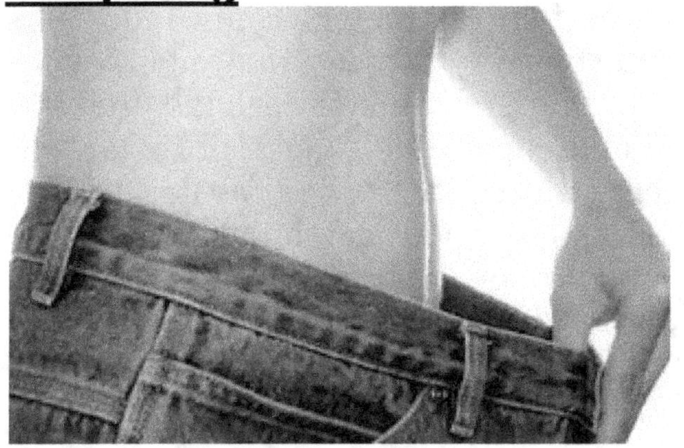

Chapter 5

KETOGENIC DIETS AND THEIR RAPID WEIGHT LOSS EFFECTS

Virtually all weight loss diets to varying degrees focus on calorie reduction or the manipulation of the intake of one of the three essential macronutrients (proteins, fats, or carbohydrates) to achieve their weight loss effects.

Ketogenic diets are a group of "high-fat, moderate protein" or "high-protein moderate fat," but very low-carbohydrate diets. The term ketogenic basically refers to the increased production of ketone bodies occasioned by the elevated rate of lipolysis (fat break down). Ketones are the acidic by-products formed during the intermediate break down of "fat" into "fatty acids" by the liver.

The first sets of ketogenic diets were designed to mimic the biochemical changes that occurred during periods of fasting, namely ketosis, acidosis, and dehydration. The diets involved the consumption of about 10-15 grams of carbohydrates per day, 1 gram of protein per kilogram bodyweight of the patient, and the remaining calories derived from fats.

Today, the promoters of ketogenic diets strongly suggest that carbohydrates especially the high glycemic index ones are the major reasons why people gain weight. Carbohydrate foods are generally metabolized to produce glucose, a form of simple sugar that is generally regarded as the preferred energy source for the body as it is a faster burning energy. Although the body can break down muscle glycogen (a mixture of glucose and water), and fat to produce energy, it however prefers to get it from high glycemic index carbohydrates from diets.

Of the macronutrients, carbohydrates are suggested to be the major cause of weight gain. This is more so because the increased intake of high glycemic index carbohydrate foods generally causes fluctuating blood sugar levels due to their fast absorption into the bloodstream, and which more often than not leads to the overproduction of insulin.

Insulin is a hormone that regulates blood glucose levels, and therefore maintenance of the energy in/energy out equation of the body which rules body weight. Excess amounts of glucose in the bloodstream causes the excessive secretion of insulin which leads to the storage of the excess glucose in the body as either glycogen in liver and muscle cells or fat in fat cells.

One aim of ketogenic diets is to reduce insulin production to its barest minimum by drastically reducing carbohydrate consumption while using fats and proteins to supplement the body's energy requirement.

Despite the ability of ketogenic diets to reduce insulin production, their main objective is ultimately aimed at inducing the state of ketosis. Ketosis can be regarded as a condition or state in which the rate of formation of ketones produced by the break down of "fat" into "fatty acids" by the liver is greater than the ability of tissues to oxidize them. Ketosis is actually a secondary state of the process of lipolysis (fat break down), and is a general side effect of low-carbohydrate diets. Ketogenic diets are therefore favorably disposed to the encouragement and promotion of ketosis.

Prolonged periods of starvation can easily induce ketosis, but it can also be deliberately induced by making use of a low-calorie or low-carbohydrate diet through the ingestion of large amounts of either fats or proteins, and drastically reduced carbohydrates. Therefore, high-fat and high-protein diets are the weight loss diets used to deliberately induce ketosis.

Essentially, ketosis is a very efficient form of energy production which does not involve the production of insulin as the body rather, burns its fat deposits for energy. Consequently, the idea of reducing carbohydrate consumption does not only reduce insulin production, but also practically forces the body to burn its fat deposit for energy, thereby making the use of ketogenic diets a very powerful way to achieve rapid weight loss.

Ketogenic diets are designed in such a way that they initially force the body to exhaust its glucose supply, and then finally switch to burning its fat deposits for energy. Subsequent food intakes after inducing the state of ketosis are meant to keep the ketosis process running by appropriately adjusting further carbohydrate consumption to provide just the basic amount of calories needed by the body.

For example, the Atkins Diet which is obviously the most popular ketogenic diet, aims to help dieters achieve what the diet calls the individual's Critical Carbohydrate Level for Maintenance (CCLM) - A carbohydrate consumption level where the dieter neither gains nor loses weight anymore.

In 2003, the Johns Hopkins treatment center came up with a modified version of the Atkins Diet protocol to treat a group of 20 children with epilepsy. After the treatment, it was observed that two-thirds experienced a significant reduction in their seizures, while 9 were able to reduce their medication dosages, and none developed kidney stones.

Furthermore, there are ongoing scientific studies by the National Institute of Health (NIH), concerning the effectiveness of the classic ketogenic diet, and the modified versions of the Atkins Diet, in helping people to lose weight, and also in the treatment of epilepsy. It is equally interesting to note that the National Institute of Neurological Disorders and Stroke (NINDS), is carrying out studies on the effect of ketogenic diets, and formulating medications that will be able to produce the same effect on weight reduction.

A KETOGENIC DIET TO LOSE WEIGHT AND FIGHT DISEASE

Obesity and metabolic diseases have become the world's biggest health problems. In fact, at least 2.8 million adults die from obesity-related causes each year.

Metabolic syndrome affects over 50 million people in the US, and can lead to a variety of health problems. To combat this, many diets have emerged, few of which are actually backed by research.

On the other hand, the benefits of the ketogenic diet are well-supported by science.

Ketogenic Diets and Weight Loss

There is strong evidence that ketogenic diets are very effective for weight loss. They can help you lose fat, preserve muscle mass, and improve many markers of disease . In fact, many studies have compared the recommended low-fat diet to a ketogenic diet for weight loss. Findings often show the ketogenic diet to be superior, even when total calorie intake is matched .

In one study, people on a ketogenic diet lost 2.2 times more weight than those on a low-calorie, low-fat diet. Triglyceride and HDL cholesterol levels also improved.

Another study compared a low-carb diet to the Diabetes UK's dietary guidelines. It found the low-carb group lost 15.2 lbs (6.9 kg), while the low-fat group lost only 4.6 lbs (2.1 kg). Over 3 months, the low-carb diet caused 3 times more weight loss.

However, there are contrasting theories for these findings. Some researchers argue that the results are simply due to a higher protein intake, and others think there is a distinct "metabolic advantage" to ketogenic diets.

Other ketogenic diet studies have found that people lose fat when food intake is not controlled or restricted. This is extremely important when applying the research to a real-life setting.

If you dislike counting calories, the data suggests a ketogenic diet is a great option for you. You can simply eliminate certain foods, and you don't have to track calories.

The ketogenic diet is an effective weight loss diet that's well-supported by evidence. It is very filling, and usually does not require calorie counting.

Mechanisms behind Ketogenic Diets and Weight Loss

Here's how ketogenic diets promote weight loss:

Higher protein intake: Some ketogenic diets lead to an increase in protein intake, which has many weight loss benefits.

Food elimination: Limiting your carb intake also limits your food options. This can noticeably reduce calorie intake, which is the key for fat loss.

Gluconeogensis: Your body converts fat and protein into carbs for fuel. This process may burn many additional calories each day.

Appetite suppressant: Ketogenic diets help you feel full. This is supported by positive changes in hunger hormones, including leptin and ghrelin.

Improved insulin sensitivity: Ketogenic diets can drastically improve insulin sensitivity, which can help improve fuel utilization and metabolism.

Decreased fat storage: Some research suggests ketogenic diets may reduce lipogenesis, the process of converting sugar into fat.

Increased fat burning: Ketogenic diets rapidly increase the amount of fat you burn during rest, daily activity and exercise.

It is very clear that a ketogenic diet can be a successful weight loss tool compared to the recommended high-carb, low-protein and low-fat diets.

A ketogenic diet may help you burn fat, reduce calorie intake, and increase feelings of fullness, compared to other weight-loss diets.

A Ketogenic Diet Can Fight Metabolic Diseases

Metabolic syndrome describes five common risk factors for obesity, type 2 diabetes, and heart disease. And they are:

High blood pressure.

Abdominal obesity (lots of belly fat).

High levels of "bad" LDL cholesterol.

Low levels of "good" HDL cholesterol.

High blood sugar levels.

Many of these risk factors can be improved or even eliminated with nutritional and lifestyle changes.

Insulin also plays an important role in diabetes and metabolic disease. Ketogenic diets are extremely effective for lowering insulin levels, especially for people with type 2 diabetes or prediabetes.

One study found that after only 2 weeks on a ketogenic diet, insulin sensitivity improved by 75%, and blood sugar dropped from 7.5 mmol/l to 6.2 mmol/l.

A 16-week study also found a 16% reduction in blood sugar levels. Additionally, 7 of the 21 participants were able to completely stop all diabetic medication.

A ketogenic diet can also have amazing effects on triglyceride levels. One study found that triglyceride evels fell from 107 to 79 mg/dL after only 4 weeks.

Ketogenic diets can improve many aspects of the metabolic syndrome, a major risk factor for obesity, type 2 diabetes, and heart disease.

The Mechanisms behind The Effects on Metabolic Disease

There are several key factors that explain the drastic effects of the ketogenic diet on markers of metabolic disease. These include:

Less carbs: A high-carb diet can constantly elevate blood sugar and insulin levels, which can lead to poor cell function and damage over time.

Decreased insulin resistance: Insulin resistance can cause health issues like inflammation, high triglyceride levels, and fat gain.

Healthy fats: The additional healthy fats you eat while on a ketogenic diet can help improve "good" HDL cholesterol levels.

Ketone bodies: Ketone bodies have some surprising benefits for health, including diseases such as cancer, Alzheimer's, and epilepsy.

Inflammation: The ketogenic diet can drastically reduce chronic inflammation, which is linked to metabolic syndrome, and various diseases.

Fat loss: This diet promotes the loss of body fat, especially unhealthy abdominal fat. Excess fat in the abdominal area is disastrous for metabolic health.

Additionally, ketogenic diets may help restore normal insulin function. Research has shown that healthy insulin function can fight inflammation, while poor insulin function can increase it.

As you can see, the combination of these factors plays an important role in health, and protection against disease.

Ketogenic diets may improve metabolic health by improving insulin function, lowering inflammation, and promoting fat loss, among others.

How to Follow a Ketogenic Diet

If you want to try a ketogenic diet, follow these basic rules:

Eliminate carbs: Check food labels, and aim for 30 grams of carbs or less per day.

Stock up on staples: Buy meat, cheese, whole eggs, nuts, oils, avocados, oily fish, and cream, as these are now staples in your diet.

Eat your veggies: Fat sources are high in calories, so base each meal on low-carb veggies to fill your plate, and help keep you feeling full.

Experiment: A ketogenic diet can still be interesting and tasty. You can even make ketogenic pasta, bread, muffins, brownies, puddings, ice cream, etc.

Build a plan: It can be hard to find low-carb meals when you're on the go. As with any diet, it is important to have a plan, and go-to snacks or meals.

Find what you love: Experiment until you find the ultimate keto diet for you.

Track progress: Take photos, measurements, and monitor your weight every 3 to 4 weeks. If progress stops, try reducing portion sizes slightly.

Replace minerals: Ketosis changes your fluid and mineral balance. For this reason, salt your food, and maybe take electrolytes or magnesium.

Try supplements: To boost the ketogenic process, you can take ketone salt supplements, MCT oil (5–10 grams twice a day) or use coconut oil regularly.

Be consistent: There is no shortcut to success. With any diet, consistency is the most important factor.

You may also wish to monitor ketone levels in either urine or blood, since these let you know whether you are keeping carb levels down sufficiently to achieve ketosis.

Base most of your meals on low-carb veggies and high-fat meats, fish or eggs.

Should You Try a Ketogenic Diet?

No single diet is suitable for everyone, especially since individual metabolism, genes, body types, lifestyles, taste buds, and personal preferences differ.

However, the ketogenic diet can work wonders for people who are overweight or at risk of metabolic syndrome.

Nevertheless, if you dislike high-fat foods, but love carbs, this diet may be hard for you to stick to. If you still like the idea of a low-carb diet, then carb cycling or a standard low-carb diet may be better options for you.

Ketogenic diets may also be used in the short-term, to help you lose fat and improve health. Yet this requires a lot of discipline, and must be followed with healthy eating.

A ketogenic diet may not be the best option for elite athletes or those wishing to build large amounts of muscle. Vegetarians or vegans may also struggle with this diet, due to the key role played by meats, eggs, fish, and dairy.

Additionally, the transition to a ketogenic diet can occasionally cause negative symptoms that are often referred to as "keto flu."

This may include poor energy and mental function, increased hunger, sleep issues, nausea, digestive discomfort, and poor exercise performance.

While this only happens rarely, it may cause some people to quit before they get started properly, especially as the first few weeks of any diet are the toughest.

Due to the very limited carb intake less than 50 grams per day ketogenic diets may also not be suitable for people who want to take the weekend off.

The ketogenic diet can provide amazing results if you stick to it. However, it may not be the best option for everyone.

In order to get the most out of a ketogenic diet, you must eat high-fat foods, and limit your carb intake to less than 30–50 grams per day.

If you stick with it, the benefits of a ketogenic diet are extremely impressive especially for health and weight loss.

Ketogenic diets can also reduce metabolic disease risk factors, and fight diseases like type 2 diabetes, and obesity.

Chapter 6

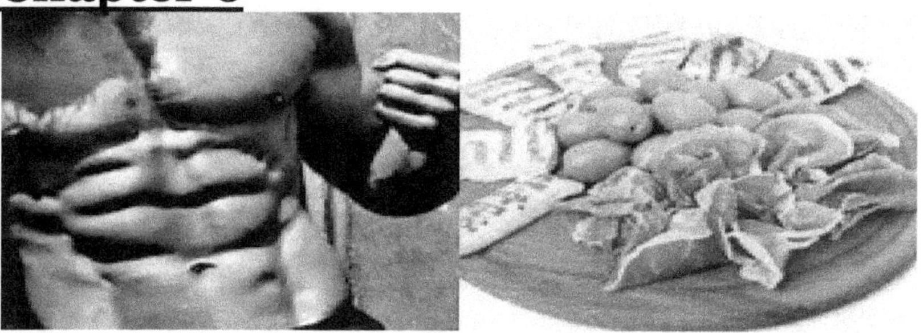

HEALTH BENEFITS OF LOW-CARB AND KETOGENIC DIETS

Low-carb diets have been controversial for decades.

They were originally demonized by fat-phobic health professionals and the media.

People believed that these diets would raise cholesterol, and cause heart disease because of the high fat content.

Since 2002, over 20 human studies have been conducted on low-carb diets.

In almost every one of those studies, low-carb diets come out ahead of the diets they are compared to.

Not only does low-carb cause more weight loss, it also leads to major improvements in most risk factors including cholesterol.

HERE ARE THE 10 PROVEN HEALTH BENEFITS OF LOW-CARB AND

KETOGENIC DIETS.

1. Low-Carb Diets Kill Your Appetite (in a Good Way)

Hunger is the single worst side effect of dieting.

It is one of the main reasons why many people feel miserable, and eventually give up on their diets.

One of the best things about eating low-carb is that it leads to an automatic reduction in appetite.

The studies consistently show that when people cut carbs and eat more protein and fat, they end up eating much fewer calories.

In fact... when researchers are comparing low-carb and low-fat diets in studies, they need to actively restrict calories in the low-fat groups to make the results comparable. When people cut carbs, their appetite tends to go down, and they often end up eating much fewer calories without trying.

2. Low-Carb Diets Lead to More Weight Loss

Cutting carbs is one of the simplest and most effective ways to lose weight.

Studies show that people on low-carb diets lose more weight, faster, than people on low-fat diets... even when the low-fat dieters are actively restricting calories.

One of the reasons for this is that low-carb diets tend to get rid of excess water from the body. Because they lower insulin levels, the kidneys start shedding excess sodium, leading to rapid weight loss in the first week or two.

In studies comparing low-carb and low-fat diets, the low-carbers sometimes lose 2-3 times as much weight, without being hungry.

 Low-carb diets appear to be particularly effective for up to 6 months, but after that the weight starts creeping back up because people give up on the diet, and start eating the same bad carbs.

It is much more appropriate to think of low-carb as a lifestyle, NOT a diet. The only way to succeed in the long-term is to stick to it.

However, some people may be able to add in healthier carbs after they have reached their goal weight.

Almost without exception, low-carb diets lead to more weight loss than the diets they are compared to, especially in the first 6 months.

3. A Greater Proportion of The Fat Lost Comes From The Abdominal Cavity

Not all fat in the body is the same. It's where that fat is stored that determines how it will affect our health, and risk of disease.

Most importantly, we have subcutaneous fat (under the skin), and we have visceral fat (in the abdominal cavity). Visceral fat is fat that tends to lodge around the organs. Having a lot of fat in that area can drive inflammation, insulin resistance, and is believed to be a leading driver of the metabolic dysfunction that is so common in Western countries today.

Low-carb diets are very effective at reducing the harmful abdominal fat.

Not only do they cause more fat loss than low-fat diets, an even greater proportion of that fat is coming from the abdominal cavity.

Over time, this should lead to a drastically reduced risk of heart disease and type 2 diabetes. A large percentage of the fat lost on low-carb diets tends to come from the harmful fat in the abdominal cavity that is known to cause serious metabolic problems.

4. Triglycerides Tend to go Way Down

Triglycerides are fat molecules. It is well known that fasting triglycerides, how much we have of them in the blood after an overnight fast, are a strong heart disease risk factor.

Perhaps counter intuitively, the main driver of elevated triglycerides is carbohydrate consumption, especially the simple sugar fructose.

When people cut carbs, they tend to have a very dramatic reduction in blood triglycerides.

Compare this to low-fat diets, which can cause triglycerides to go up in many cases.

Low-carb diets are very effective at lowering blood triglycerides, which are fat molecules in the blood, and a well-known risk factor for heart disease.

5. Increased Levels of HDL (the "good") Cholesterol

High Density Lipoprotein (HDL) is often called the "good" cholesterol.

It's actually wrong to call it "cholesterol"... all cholesterol molecules are the same.

HDL and LDL refer to the lipoproteins that carry cholesterol around in the blood. Whereas LDL carries cholesterol from the liver, and to the rest of the body, HDL carries cholesterol away from the body and to the liver, where it can be reused or excreted.

It is well known that the higher your levels of HDL, the lower your risk of heart disease will be. One of the best ways to increase HDL levels is to eat fat... and low-carb diets include a lot of fat.

Therefore, it is not surprising to see that HDL levels increase dramatically on low-carb diets, while they tend to increase only moderately or even go down on low-fat diets.

The Triglycerides: HDL ratio is another very strong predictor of heart disease risk. The higher it is, the greater your risk of heart disease is.

By lowering triglycerides and raising HDL levels, low-carb diets lead to a major improvement in this ratio.

Low-carb diets tend to be high in fat, which leads to an impressive increase in blood levels of HDL, often referred to as the "good" cholesterol.

6. Reduced Blood Sugar and Insulin Levels: With a Major Improvement in Type 2 Diabetes

When we eat carbs, they are broken down into simple sugars (mostly glucose) in the digestive tract. From there, they enter the bloodstream and elevate blood sugar levels.

Because high blood sugars are toxic, the body responds with a hormone called insulin, which tells the cells to bring the glucose into the cells, and to start burning or storing it.

For people who are healthy, the quick insulin response tends to minimize the blood sugar "spike" in order to prevent it from harming us.

However, many people have major problems with this system. They have what is called insulin resistance, which means that the cells don't "see" the insulin, and therefore it is harder for the body to bring the blood sugar into the cells.

This can lead to a disease called type 2 diabetes, when the body fails to secrete enough insulin to lower the blood sugar after meals. This disease is very common today, afflicting about 300 million people worldwide.

There is actually a very simple solution to this problem... by cutting carbohydrates, you remove the need for all of that insulin. Both blood sugars and insulin go way down.

In one study in type 2 diabetics, 95.2% had managed to reduce or eliminate their glucose-lowering medication within 6 months.

If you are currently on blood sugar lowering medication, then talk to your doctor before making any changes to your carbohydrate intake, because your dosage may need to be adjusted in order to prevent hypoglycemia.

The best way to lower blood sugar and insulin levels is to reduce carbohydrate consumption. This is also a very effective way to treat, and possibly even reverse type II diabetes.

7. Blood Pressure Tends to go down

Having elevated blood pressure (hypertension) is an important risk factor for many diseases. This includes heart disease, stroke, kidney failure, and many others. Low-carb diets are an effective way to reduce blood pressure, which should lead to a reduced risk of these diseases, and help you live longer.

Studies show that reducing carbs leads to a significant reduction in blood pressure, which should lead to a reduced risk of many common diseases.

8. Low-Carb Diets Are The Most Effective Treatment Known Against Metabolic Syndrome

The metabolic syndrome is a medical condition that is highly associated with the risk of diabetes and heart disease.

It is actually a collection of symptoms such as:

Abdominal obesity

Elevated blood pressure

Elevated fasting blood sugar levels

High triglycerides

Low HDL levels

The good news is, all five symptoms improve dramatically on a low-carb diet.

Unfortunately, the government and major health organization still recommend a low-fat diet for this purpose, which is pretty much useless because it does nothing to address the underlying metabolic problem.

Low-carb diets effectively reverse all 5 key symptoms of the metabolic syndrome, a serious condition known to predispose people to heart disease and type 2 diabetes.

9. Low-Carb Diets Improve The Pattern of LDL Cholesterol

Low Density Lipoprotein (LDL) is often referred to as the "bad" cholesterol (again, it is actually a protein).

It is known that people who have high LDL are much more likely to have heart attacks. However, what scientists have now learned is that the type of LDL matters. Not all of them are equal.

In this regard, the size of the particles is important. People who have mostly small particles have a high risk of heart disease, while people who have mostly large particles have a low risk.

It turns out that low-carb diets actually turn the LDL particles from small to large, while reducing the number of LDL particles floating around in the bloodstream.

When you eat a low-carb diet, your LDL particles change from small (bad) LDL to large LDL - which is benign. Cutting carbs may also reduce the number of LDL particles floating around in the bloodstream.

10. Low-Carb Diets Are Therapeutic For Several Brain Disorders

It is often claimed that glucose is necessary for the brain... and it's true.

Some part of the brain can only burn glucose. That's why the liver produces glucose out of protein if we don't eat any carbs. But a large part of the brain can also burn ketones, which are formed during starvation or when carbohydrate intake is very low.

This is the mechanism behind the ketogenic diet, which has been used for decades to treat epilepsy in children who don't respond to drug treatment.

In many cases, this diet can cure children of epilepsy. In one study, over half of the children on a ketogenic diet had a greater than 50% reduction in seizures. Sixteen percent of the children became seizure free.

Very low-carb/ketogenic diets are now being studied for other brain disorders as well, including Alzheimer's disease, and Parkinson's disease.

Chapter 7

Ketogenic
Diet for Epilepsy

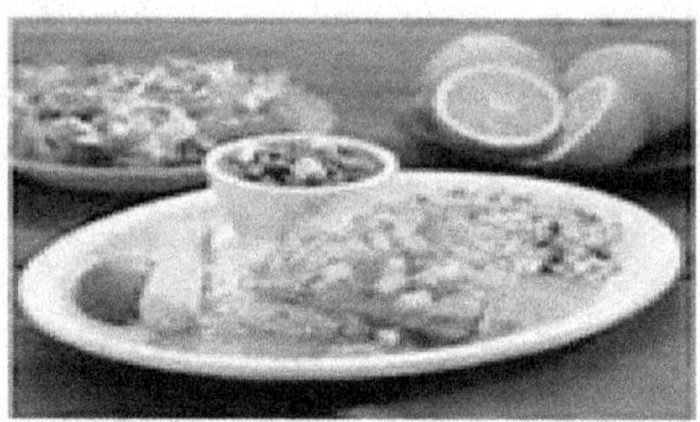

KETOGENIC DIET FOR EPILEPTIC CHILDREN

Could the solution to your child's epilepsy be a diet loaded with butter, cream, oils, and mayo? It might sound weird, and maybe not so appetizing, but the ketogenic diet is real, and in many kids, it works.

But the super high-fat, super low-carb ketogenic diet is not for everyone. It's strict and complicated, and not really "healthy" in the normal sense. If you're considering it, you need to think through how it will affect your child's life, and the impact on the whole family.

Who Should Think about Trying the Ketogenic Diet?

The ketogenic diet has been curbing seizures since it was first developed in the 1920s. About half of kids who follow it have a big drop in how many episodes they get. As many as 1 in 7 stop having seizures completely.

The diet helps with many types of epilepsy, but works especially well with Lennox-Gastaut syndrome, myoclonic astatic epilepsy (Doose syndrome), and others. It can also help people of any age, but it's mostly used in babies and children. That's mainly because teens and adults have so much trouble sticking to it.

Because the ketogenic diet is so demanding, doctors usually only recommend it if a child has already tried two or three medications, and they haven't worked.

When the diet works, kids can often lower their medication doses or stop taking them all together. According to research, most kids who stay on the ketogenic diet for at least 2 years have a good chance of becoming seizure free even after they go back to eating normally.

What Foods Can Your Child Eat?

Your child's diet will have a lot of fat. To put it in perspective, in a healthy diet for kids, about 25% to 40% of calories come from fat. In the ketogenic diet, about 80% to 90% of calories come from fat.

So your child's meals are loaded with fats while portions of protein and carbs are small. In the typical ketogenic diet, kids get three to four times as much fat at each meal compared to carbs and protein combined.

What does that mean in practice? Most high-carb foods like bread, pasta, sweets, and more are off the menu.

How Does It Work?

Even though it's been around for 1 hundred years, we still don't know. Many experts believed it had to do with a process called ketosis. That's where the diet's name comes from. Ketosis happens when your body runs out of carbohydrates to burn for energy, and burns fat instead.

But now many experts aren't sure if ketosis has anything to do with why the diet works. It may be related to some other effect we don't understand.

What to Expect

The ketogenic diet is not something you try out casually. It's a big commitment, and starting it on your own is risky. You and your child need to work closely with a team of experts.

Prepare for a few days in the hospital. Doctors often want to keep an eye on kids when they start the diet to make sure they're doing OK.

Work closely with a dietitian. The ketogenic diet is tailored to each child. So a dietitian will give you detailed information on exactly what your child can eat and how much. Since the ketogenic diet is low in important nutrients, your child will probably need supplements of calcium, vitamin D, iron, folic acid, and others.

Watch out for carbs in everything. Tiny amounts of carbs show up in unexpected places, like toothpaste.

See the doctor often. Your child will need regular checkups every 1 to 3 months at first. The doctor will chart his or her growth and weight, test her blood and urine, and decide whether to tweak the diet or medication dose.

Stick with the diet for a few months at least. If it works, you should notice fewer seizures by then -- or even sooner. If the diet doesn't help, your child will gradually return to a normal eating plan. If he or she stops the ketogenic diet suddenly, it could trigger seizures.

What Are the Side Effects?

Right after your child starts the diet, he or she may feel tired. Other side effects include:

Constipation

Kidney stones

Slow growth and low weight

Weak bones (which may be more likely to break)

High cholesterol

If your child has side effects, tell her doctor. You may be able to treat them with changes to his or her diet, or medication.

If the side effects are too much for your child, ask the doctor about other epilepsy diets, like the modified Atkins diet, and the low glycemic index treatment diet. They can be a little easier to handle.

Is the Ketogenic Diet Right for Your Child?

You have to decide if your family is ready for the ketogenic diet. You'll need to change the food you have in your home, and the meals you eat. That can be tricky if you have other kids in the family.

All caregivers for your child from babysitters to teachers have to understand the diet, and be on board, too. Even a little cheating on the food plan could trigger a seizure.

If you think you're up for it, talk to your child's doctor. Going "keto" is never easy, but for many kids, it can be a big success.

Chapter 8

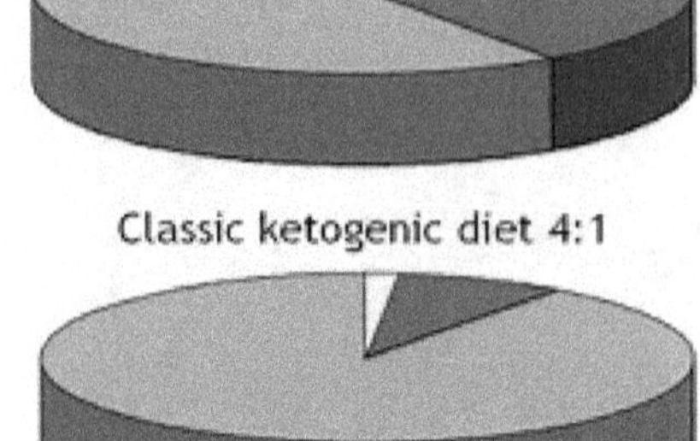

Classic ketogenic diet 4:1

WHAT IS KETOSIS, AND IS IT HEALTHY

Ketosis is a natural metabolic state. It involves the body producing ketone bodies out of fat, and using them for energy instead of carbs.

You can get into ketosis by following a very low-carb, high-fat ketogenic diet.

In addition to fast weight loss, ketosis may have several health benefits, such as reduced seizures in epileptic children.

Ketosis is quite complex, but this chapter explains what it is and how it can benefit you.

What is Ketosis?

Ketosis is a metabolic state in which fat provides most of the fuel for the body.

It occurs when there is limited access to glucose (blood sugar), which is the preferred fuel source for many cells in the body.

Ketosis is most often associated with ketogenic, and very low-carb diets. It also happens during pregnancy, infancy, fasting, and starvation.

To go into ketosis, people generally need to eat fewer than 50 grams of carbs per day, and sometimes as little as 20 grams per day.

This requires removing certain food items from your diet, such as grains, candy, and sugary soft drinks. You also have to cut back on legumes, potatoes, and fruit.

When eating a very low-carb diet, levels of the hormone insulin go down, and fatty acids are released from body fat stores in large amounts.

Many of these fatty acids are transferred to the liver, where they are oxidized and turned into ketones (or ketone bodies). These molecules can provide energy for the body.

Unlike fatty acids, ketones can cross the blood-brain barrier, and provide energy for the brain in the absence of glucose.

Ketosis is a metabolic state where ketones become the main sources of energy for the body and brain. This happens when carb intake and insulin levels are very low.

Ketones Can Supply Energy for the Brain

It is a common misunderstanding that the brain doesn't function without dietary carbs. It's true that glucose is preferred, and that there are some cells in the brain that can only use glucose for fuel.

However, a large portion of your brain can also use ketones for energy, such as during starvation or when your diet is low in carbs.

In fact, after only three days of starvation, the brain gets 25% of its energy from ketones. During long-term starvation, this number rises to about 60%.

In addition, your body can use protein to produce the little glucose the brain still requires during ketosis. This process is called gluconeogenesis.

Ketosis and gluconeogenesis are perfectly capable of fulfilling the brain's energy needs.

How Low-Carb and Ketogenic Diets Boost Brain Health

When the brain isn't getting enough glucose, it can use ketones for energy. The little glucose it still needs can be produced from protein.

Ketosis is NOT the Same as Ketoacidosis

People often confuse ketosis and ketoacidosis. While ketosis is part of normal metabolism, ketoacidosis is a dangerous metabolic condition that can be fatal if left untreated.

In ketoacidosis, the bloodstream is flooded with extremely high levels of glucose (blood sugar), and ketones. When this happens, the blood becomes acidic, which is seriously harmful. Ketoacidosis is most often associated with uncontrolled type 1 diabetes. It may also occur in people with type 2 diabetes, although this is less common.

In addition, severe alcohol abuse may lead to ketoacidosis.

Ketosis is a natural metabolic state, while ketoacidosis is a serious medical condition, and most often seen in uncontrolled type 1 diabetes.

Effects on Epilepsy

Epilepsy is a brain disorder characterized by recurring seizures.

It is a very common neurological condition, affecting around 70 million people worldwide.

For the majority of patients, anti-seizure medications can help control the seizures. However, around 30% of patients continue to have seizures despite using these medications.

In the early 1920's, the ketogenic diet was introduced as a treatment for epilepsy in people who don't respond to drug treatment.

It has primarily been used in children, with some studies showing remarkable benefits. Many epileptic children have had massive reductions in seizures on a ketogenic diet, and some have even seen complete remission.

Ketogenic diets can effectively reduce epileptic seizures, especially in epileptic children who don't respond to conventional treatment.

Effects on Weight Loss

The ketogenic diet is a popular weight loss diet that is well-supported by science. In fact, many studies have found that ketogenic diets lead to much greater weight loss than low-fat diets.

One study reported 2.2 times more weight loss for people on a ketogenic diet, compared to those on a low-fat, calorie-restricted diet.

Also, people tend to feel less hungry, and more full on a ketogenic diet, which is attributed to ketosis. For this reason, it is generally not necessary to count calories on this diet.

Studies show that ketogenic diets lead to more weight loss than low-fat diets. In addition, people feel less hungry, and more fullfilling.

Other Health Benefits of Ketosis

Ketosis and ketogenic diets may also have other therapeutic effects. They are now being studied as a treatment for a wide variety of conditions such as:

Heart disease - Reducing carbs to achieve ketosis may improve heart disease risk factors like blood triglycerides, total cholesterol and HDL cholesterol.

Type 2 diabetes - The diet may improve insulin sensitivity by up to 75%, and some diabetics are able to reduce or even stop diabetes medication.

Metabolic syndrome - Ketogenic diets can improve all major symptoms of metabolic syndrome, including high triglycerides, excess belly fat, and elevated blood pressure.

Alzheimer's disease - A ketogenic diet may have benefits for patients with Alzheimer's disease.

Cancer - Some studies suggest that ketogenic diets may aid in cancer therapy, possibly by helping to "starve" cancer cells of glucose.

Parkinson's disease - A small study found that symptoms of Parkinson's disease improved after 28 days on a ketogenic diet.

Acne - There is some evidence that this diet may reduce the severity and progression of acne.

Ketosis and ketogenic diets may help with a number of chronic diseases, including metabolic syndrome, type 2 diabetes, and Alzheimer's.

Does Ketosis Have Any Negative Health Effects?

There are a few potential side effects you may experience from ketosis, and ketogenic diets. These include headache, fatigue, constipation, high cholesterol levels and bad breath.

However, most of the symptoms are temporary, and should disappear within a few days or weeks.

Also, some epileptic children have developed kidney stones on the diet .

Although extremely rare, there have been a few cases of breastfeeding women developing ketoacidosis likely triggered by a low-carb or ketogenic diet.

People who are taking blood sugar lowering drugs should consult with a doctor before trying a ketogenic diet, because the diet may reduce the need for medication.

Sometimes ketogenic diets are low in fiber. For this reason, it is a good idea to make sure to eat plenty of high-fiber, low-carb vegetables. All that being said, ketosis is generally safe for healthy people.

Nevertheless, it is not for everyone. Some people may feel great and full of energy in ketosis, while others feel miserable.

Ketosis is safe for most people. However, some people may experience side effects, including bad breath, headaches, and constipation.

Signs and Symptoms That You're in Ketosis

The ketogenic diet is a popular, effective way to lose weight and improve health.

When followed correctly, this low-carb, high-fat diet will raise blood ketone levels.

These provide a new fuel source for your cells, and cause most of the unique health benefits of this diet.

On a ketogenic diet, your body undergoes many biological adaptions, including a reduction in insulin, and increased fat breakdown.

When this happens, your liver starts producing large amounts of ketones to supply energy for your brain.

However, it can often be hard to know whether you're "in ketosis" or not.

Here are 10 common signs and symptoms of ketosis, both positive and negative.

1. Bad Breath

People often report bad breath once they reach full ketosis.

It's actually a common side effect. Many people on ketogenic diets and similar diets, such as the Atkins diet, report that their breath takes on a fruity smell.

This is caused by elevated ketone levels. The specific culprit is acetone, a ketone that exits the body in your urine and breath.

While this breath may be less than ideal for your social life, it can be a positive sign for your diet. Many ketogenic dieters brush their teeth several times per day, or use sugar-free gum to solve the issue.

If you're using gum or other alternatives like sugar-free drinks, check the label for carbs. These may raise your blood sugar levels, and reduce ketone levels. The bad breath usually goes away after some time on the diet. It is not a permanent thing. The ketone acetone is partly expelled by your breath, which can cause bad or fruity-smelling breath on a ketogenic diet.

2. Weight Loss

Ketogenic diets, along with normal low-carb diets, are highly effective for losing weight.

As dozens of weight loss studies have shown, you will likely experience both short- and long-term weight loss when switching to a ketogenic diet.

Fast weight loss can occur during the first week. While some people believe this to be fat loss, it is primarily stored carbs and water being used up.

After the initial rapid drop in water weight, you should continue to lose body fat consistently as long as you stick to the diet and remain in a calorie deficit.

Fast weight loss commonly occurs when you start a ketogenic diet, and severely restrict carbohydrates.

3. Increased Ketones in the Blood

One of the hallmarks of a ketogenic diet is a reduction in blood sugar levels, and an increase in ketones.

As you progress further into a ketogenic diet, you will start to burn fat, and ketones as the main fuel sources.

The most reliable and accurate method of measuring ketosis is to measure your blood ketone levels using a specialized meter.

It measures your ketone levels by calculating the amount of beta-hydroxybutyrate (BHB) in your blood. This is one of the primary ketones present in the bloodstream.

According to some experts on the ketogenic diet, nutritional ketosis is defined as blood ketones ranging from 0.5–3.0 mmol/L per meter.

Measuring ketones in the blood is the most accurate way of testing, and is used in most research studies. However, the main downside is that it requires a small pinprick to draw blood from the finger .

A test kit also costs around $30–$40, and then an additional $5 per test. For this reason, most people will just perform one test per week, or every two weeks. Testing blood ketone levels with a monitor is the most accurate way to measure whether you are in ketosis or not.

4. Increased Ketones in the Breath or Urine

Another way to measure blood ketone levels is a breath analyzer.

It monitors acetone, one of the three main ketones present in your blood during ketosis.

This helps give you an idea about your body's ketone levels, since more acetone leaves the body when you are in nutritional ketosis.

The use of acetone breath analyzers has been shown to be fairly accurate, but less accurate than the blood monitor method.

Another good technique is to measure the presence of ketones in your urine on a daily basis with special indicator strips.

These also measure ketone excretion through the urine, and can be a quick and cheap method to assess your ketone levels daily. However, they are not considered very reliable.

You can measure your ketone levels with a breath analyzer or urine strips. However, they are not as accurate as a blood monitor.

5. Appetite Suppression

Many people report decreased hunger while following a ketogenic diet.

However, it's been suggested the hunger reduction may be due to an increased protein and vegetable intake, along with alterations to your body's hunger hormones.

The ketones themselves may affect the brain to reduce appetite.

A ketogenic diet can significantly reduce appetite and hunger. If you feel full and don't need to eat as often as before, then you may be in ketosis.

6. Increased Focus and Energy

People often report brain fog, tiredness, and feeling sick when first starting a very low-carb diet. This is termed the "low carb flu" or "keto flu." However, long-term ketogenic dieters often report increased focus, and energy.

When you start a low-carb diet, your body must adapt to burning more fat for fuel, instead of carbs.

When you get into ketosis, a large part of the brain starts burning ketones instead of glucose. It can take a few days or weeks for this to start working properly.

Ketones are an extremely potent fuel source for the brain. They even have been tested in a medical setting to treat brain diseases, and conditions such as concussion and memory loss .

Therefore, it comes as no surprise that long-term ketogenic dieters often report increased clarity, and improved brain function .

Eliminating carbs can also help control and stabilize blood sugar levels. This may further increase focus and improve brain function.

Many long-term ketogenic dieters report improved brain function, and more stable energy levels, likely due to the rise in ketones, and more stable blood sugar levels.

7. Short-Term Fatigue

The initial switch to a ketogenic diet can be one of the biggest issues for new dieters. Its well-known side effects can include weakness and fatigue.

These often cause people to quit the diet before they get into full ketosis and reap many of the long-term benefits.

These side effects are natural. After several decades of running on a carb-heavy fuel system, your body is forced to adapt to a new system.

As you might expect, this switch does not occur overnight. It normally requires 7–30 days before you are in full ketosis.

To help reduce fatigue during this switch, you may want to take electrolyte supplements.

Electrolytes are often lost because of the rapid reduction in your body's water content, and the elimination of processed foods that may contain added salt.

When adding these supplements, try to obtain 2,000–4,000 mg of sodium, 1,000 mg of potassium, and 300 mg of magnesium per day.

Initially, you may suffer from tiredness and low energy. This will pass once your body becomes adapted to running on fat and ketones.

8. Short-Term Decreases in Performance

As discussed above, removing carbs can lead to general tiredness at first. This includes an initial decrease in exercise performance.

It is primarily caused by the reduction in your muscles' glycogen stores, which provide the main, and most efficient fuel source for all forms of high-intensity exercise.

After several weeks, many ketogenic dieters state that their performance returns to normal. In certain types of ultra-endurance sports and events, a ketogenic diet could actually be beneficial.

There are also some further benefits, primarily an increased ability to burn more fat during exercise.

One famous study found that athletes who had switched to a ketogenic diet burned as much as 230% more fat when they exercised, compared to athletes who were not on a ketogenic diet.

While it is unlikely that a ketogenic diet can maximize performance for elite athletes, once you become fat-adapted it should be sufficient for general exercise and recreational sports.

Short-term decreases in performance can occur. However, they tend to improve again after the initial adaptation phase is over.

9. Digestive Issues

A ketogenic diet generally involves a major change in the types of foods you eat. Digestive issues such as constipation and diarrhea are pretty common side effects in the beginning. Most of these issues should subside after the transition period, but it may be important to be mindful of different foods that may be causing digestive issues.

Also, make sure to eat plenty of healthy low-carb veggies. They are low in carbs, but still contain plenty of fiber.

You might experience digestive issues such as constipation when you first switch to a ketogenic diet.

10. Insomnia

One big issue for many ketogenic dieters is sleep, especially when they first change their diet. A lot of people report insomnia or waking up at night when they first reduce their carbs drastically.

However, this usually improves in a matter of weeks. Many long-term ketogenic dieters claim that they sleep better than before after adapting to the diet. Poor sleep and insomnia is a common symptom during the initial stages of ketosis. This usually improves after a few weeks.

Chapter 9

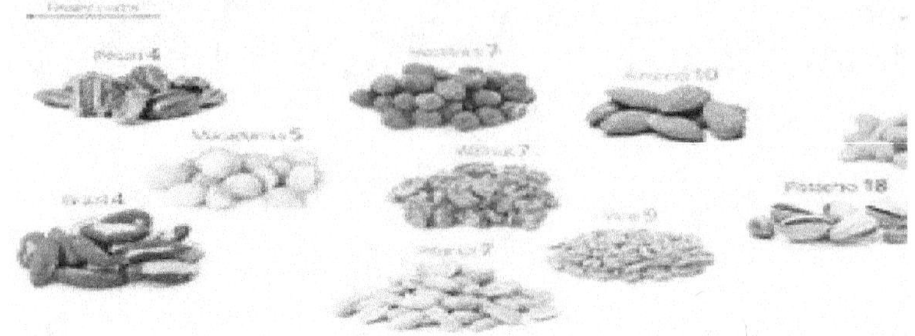

10 FOODS YOU MUST HAVE IN YOUR KITCHEN

The ketogenic diet is a very successful weight-loss program. It utilizes high fat and low carbohydrate ingredients in order to burn fat instead of glucose. Many people are familiar with the Atkins diet, but the keto plan restricts carbs even more.

Because we are surrounded by fast food restaurants and processed meals, it can be a challenge to avoid carb-rich foods, but proper planning can help.

Plan menus and snacks at least a week ahead of time, so you aren't caught with only high carb meal choices. Immerse yourself in the keto lifestyle, find your favorite recipes, and stick with them.

There are a few items that are a must of a keto diet. Be sure to have these items on hand:

Eggs - Used in omelets, quiches (yes, heavy cream is legal on keto!), hard boiled as a snack, low carb pizza crust, and more; if you like eggs, you have a great chance of success on this diet.

Bacon - Do I need a reason? Breakfast, salad garnish, burger topper, BLT's (no bread of course; try a BLT in a bowl, tossed in mayo).

Cream cheese - Dozens of recipes, pizza crusts, main dishes, and desserts.

Shredded cheese - Sprinkle over taco meat in a bowl, made into tortilla chips in the microwave, salad toppers, low-carb pizza and enchiladas.

Lots of romaine and spinach - Fill up on the green veggies; have plenty on hand for a quick salad when hunger pains hit.

EZ-Sweets liquid sweetener - Use a couple of drops in place of sugar; this artificial sweetener is the most natural and easiest to use.

Cauliflower - Fresh or frozen bags you can eat this low-carb veggie by itself, tossed in olive oil and baked, mashed in fake potatoes, chopped/shredded and used in place of rice under main dishes, in low-carb and keto pizza crusts, and much more.

Frozen chicken tenders - Have a large bag on hand; thaw quickly and grill, saute, mix with veggies, and top with garlic sauce in a low carb flatbread, use in Chicken piccata, chicken alfredo, tacos, enchiladas, Indian Butter chicken, and more.

Ground beef - Make a big burger top with all sorts of things from cheese, to sauteed mushrooms, to grilled onions... or crumble and cook with taco seasoning, and use in provolone cheese taco shells; throw in a dish with lettuce, avocado, cheese, sour cream for a tortilla-less taco salad.

Almonds (plain or flavored) - These are a tasty and healthy snack; however, be sure to count them as you eat, because the carbs DO add up. .Flavors include habanero, coconut, salt and vinegar, and more.

The keto plan is a versatile and interesting way to lose weight, with lots of delicious food choices. .Keep these 10 items stocked in your fridge, freezer, and you'll be ready to throw together some delicious keto meals, and snacks at a moment's notice.

THE BENEFITS OF MIXING MCT OIL INTO YOUR KETOGENIC DIET PLAN

Most people talk about what they must haves. If you're driving a high end car, you must have the top of the line motor oil coursing through its cylinders. If you're competing at a high level in a track competition, state of the art running shoes are a must have. When you're celebrating a huge quarter at the office, the finest bourbon is a must have. I would submit to you, that if you're serious about a ketogenic lifestyle, MCT Oil is a must have.

MCT Oil provides a heavy dose of the very fuels that turn your body into - and keep it - a fat burning machine. Unlike LCTs, MCTs bypass much of the digestion process that others fats go through, and acts in an almost carb-like manner in how they're sent directly to the liver, where they are used for energy.

There are many reasons why MCT makes perfect sense for your Ketogenic Diet, but help you understand how they can play an essential role in your nutrition, we've some of the main benefits of MCT Oil in your Ketogenic Diet plan.

MCT OIL HELPS YOU GET INTO KETOSIS FASTER

As was said earlier, MCTs go to your liver, and act in a "carb-like" manner that LCTs do not have the ability to do. This means that you can theoretically kickstart Ketosis by following these steps:

1. Fast with no breakFAST

If you've been out of Ketosis for awhile and you want to efficiently get back into a fat burning state, a mix of fasting and MCT Oil will do the job. Just eat a very low carb dinner, or even skip dinner, and then wake up and don't eat breakfast! Instead, drink a cup of coffee, and put a tablespoon or two of MCT Oil into your coffee, and head out!

The shot of MCT, plus the already fasted state of your body will have you back into Ketosis quicker than if you tried to just slowly eat your way back into Ketosis (i.e. nutritional Ketosis). It's also worth adding that the energy you get from the MCT Oil, and the coffee will be unlike what you were used to: the MCTs provide a prolonged energy that isn't comparable to energy derived from glycogen.

2. Meal replacement with MCT Oil

Another benefit that comes from using MCT Oil in your Ketogenic Diet plan is using it as a meal replacement.

This somewhat resembles the previous point of fasting with MCT Oil, but the difference is that you're still eating other regular Ketogenic meals, except your replacing (at least) one of those meals with some MCT Oil.

One of the benefits of MCT Oil is its ability to satiate your appetite. So while it sounds initially scary to just depend a few tablespoons of oil for a meal replacement, your body will become accustomed as you do it more and more. The MCTs will act as replacement for what's normally there (glycogen), and your fierce-badger-hunger cravings will lessen.

In our fast paced, 21st century lifestyle, the benefits of being able to remain in Ketosis while only slurping a few tablespoons of MCTs cannot be overstated.

3. Ramp up your Ketogenic dishes with MCT

MCT Oil's versatility is amazing. Let's say you're already in Ketosis, but you're about to eat a salad for your daily carbs, and you want to keep it 100 on the Keto life. It's easy! Just use MCT for a base to your dressing, and you can rest assured that you'll still be burning fat after you've downed your greens!

Another way to use MCTs in your favorite Ketogenic meals is to use it as a replacement for regular oil in baking! There's a whole ocean of Keto baking recipes out there, so why not double down and use MCT instead of regular coconut oil.

But what if you're not baking? What if you're out for a jog, and you want to implement the energy efficiency of MCT Oil? How about a nice Keto "sports drink." All you have to do is get your water, and then squeeze in some lemon juice, and you'll have a healthier, non-sugary sports drink for long workouts in the sun.

There are many ways to skin a cat, and there's also many ways to amplify your Ketogenic Diet. MCTs are essential to your body transforming into a fat burning machine. Unfortunately, you're not always going to be able to get the proper amounts from a diet alone - you'll need a boost, and MCT Oil is that boost you are looking for.

Life is full of "must haves," and your diet does not fall out of the realm of this mantra. If you want to live a truly Ketogenic lifestyle, you're going to have invest in the right fuels, and implement them in the most efficient ways possible. So what's the benefit of MCT to your Ketogenic Diet plan? The answer is efficiency. An efficient diet, which feeds an efficient lifestyle that will ultimately give you more time to do the things you love.

Chapter 10

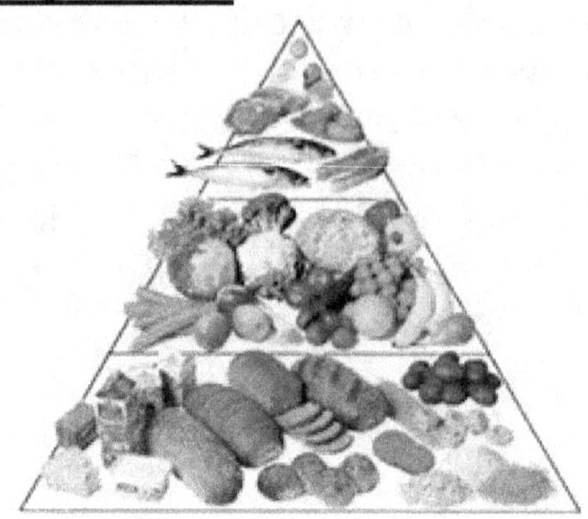

25 KETO RECIPES

Trying new diets can be tough, having to avoid all those things you love to eat, and new ingredients to buy. It's enough to drive anyone bonkers. But there's one way of eating that's been gaining momentum lately, the ketogenic, or "keto," diet, and its keto recipes.

The ketogenic diet is one of the most effective that I've come across, and one of the more straightforward to follow.   In a nutshell, when you're on a keto diet, you eat a very low-carb, high-fat diet. That means goodbye pasta and bread, and say hello cheese and oils. It's pretty much the opposite of what we've been taught our entire lives. But it works if you follow the keto diet food list.

What makes the keto diet work so well is that, with little glucose from carbohydrates in our bodies, we have to burn other fat for energy. The keto diet can cause the body to burn fat quickly.

If you're not trying to lose weight, the keto diet might appeal to you as well. By limiting sugars and processed grains, you lower your risk of type 2 diabetes. Eating an array of heart-healthy fats, like nuts, olive oil and fish, can decrease your risk of heart disease. And while some people stick to a super strict keto diet, with 75 percent of their diet coming from fat, 20 percent from protein, and just 5 from carbs, even a less intense modified version can help you reap the keto diet's benefits.

But eating keto doesn't mean eating just any kind of fat or stuffing your face with ice cream. Instead, it's about mindfully choosing foods that are high in healthy fats and low in carbs. If you're not sure where to begin, have no fear. There are some really delicious, good-for-you keto recipes out there that are begging to be eaten.

KETO RECIPES INGREDIENTS

1. Avocado and Eggs Fat Bombs

Looking for a way to add in extra healthy fats and protein to your diet? These fat bombs have you covered. They're made from avocados, which are loaded with monounsaturated fats and vitamins, along with protein-packed eggs. Use homemade mayonnaise to make these extra healthy.

2. Best Keto Bread

Do keto recipes include bread? Yes! Satisfy your bread cravings with this keto-friendly recipe. This loaf is made with gluten-free, low-carb almond flour that's light and fluffy thanks to a great tip about separating the eggs.

3. Cauliflower Crusted Grilled Cheese Sandwiches

Get a load of veggies and cheese with this ingenious keto recipe. You'll dry out the cauliflower, then bake it into "bread" slices that get stacked with cheese; use a high-quality, organic cheddar here. It's worth it.

4. Chicken Pad Thai

This low-carb chicken pad thai is one of the best keto recipes for replacing Asian takeout. It's got all of the flavors that come with normal pad thai, like ginger, crushed peanuts, tamari and chicken, but all served up on spiralized zucchini instead of carb-heavy noodles. Best of all, you'll have this one on the table in just 30 minutes.

5. Chocolate Fat Bombs

The beauty about the keto diet is that sometimes you just haven't eaten enough fat in the day, and so you chow down on "fat bombs" to make up the deficit. These chocolate bombs are one of the yummiest ways to do that. Just mix butter, cream cheese, cacao powder, and a small amount of sweetener for some chocolatey goodness that'll do your body good.

6. Cinnamon Butter Bombs

Grass-fed butter is a terrific way to add quality fat into your diet. Plus, it's full of health benefits: This type of butter is anti-inflammatory, better for your heart than standard butter and full of MCTs, which boost your immune system.

But if you're not ready to eat a stick of butter solo, just make these cinnamon bombs. By simply adding vanilla extract, cinnamon and sweetener to your butter, and letting them cool, you have a little treat that's full of healthy fats and tastes like frosting.

7. Coconut Oil Mayonnaise

You'll often find keto recipes calling for mayonnaise. But why waste your money on store-bought varieties that are filled with ingredients like canola oil when you can make your own at home? You'll be surprised by how easy mayo is to whip up at home, and it lasts until your eggs expire.

8. Creamy Cauliflower Mash and Keto Gravy

Potatoes and gravy are total comfort food, and luckily there's a keto version. These are made with cauliflower, which is quite low-carb, particularly when compared to potatoes. Made with cream, butter, rosemary and parmesan, this mash is creamy, full of flavor, and smooth. You'll finish it all off with a stock-based gravy, that would be perfect on a roast, too.

9. Crustless Spinach Quiche

Fortunately, keto recipes can include quiche. This one looks fancy, but it's effortless to put together. With just a handful of ingredients, including high-protein eggs, lots of cheese and zero grains, it's awesome for serving at brunch.

10. Easy Cheesy Zucchini Gratin

Everything is better with cheese including zucchini. This low-carb, high-cheese gratin replaces potatoes with fresh green zucchini, and makes a perfect side dish or light main dish.

11. Easy Crockpot Chicken Stew

This keto recipe is a double win. Not only is it low-carb and creamy, but you just dump all the ingredients into the crockpot, and let it works its magic. With herbs like rosemary, oregano, and thyme all making an appearance, and juiced chicken thighs as the protein, this is one stew you'll make over and over again.

12. Fathead Nachos

You'll begin by making the fat head tortilla chips first. Did I mention you'll use two types of cheese for this step? Delicious. Next, you'll load them up with a meaty sauce and finish them off with your favorite toppings, like guac, salsa or sour cream. While these make a delicious snack, they're frankly filling enough to share as a meal.

13. Gluten-Free Cauliflower Mac and Cheese

Can you really make a gluten-free, low-carb macaroni and cheese that tastes good? The verdict after trying this keto recipe is yes! Cauliflower, that magical vegetable, stands in for macaroni here, but it's really the cheese and kefir that make this one stand out.

Kefir is a fermented milk-like drink that's rich in probiotics and great for your gut. We'll also use sheep and goat milk cheese, which is a smart option for people who are lactose intolerant or just want to vary up their cheese. You'll love serving this, and your family will love eating it.

14. Jalapeno Cheddar Burgers

Why top a burger with cheese when you can stuff it instead? You'll envelop each patty (your choice of turkey or beef) with a mixture of cheeses, garlic and jalapeño, then grill or broil to perfection. Each bite is better than the last.

15. Keto Blueberry Muffins

These keto muffins are a bit labor intensive, but they're a delicious way to kick off the day. Made with coconut flour, butter, cream cheese and fresh blueberries, you'll never believe they're gluten-free when you see how light and fluffy they are.   A crowd favorite!

16. Keto Oatmeal

Hemp hearts are rich in fat, and oatmeal is a great way to use the healthy ingredient. This collection of hemp-based oatmeal recipes has seven different variations to get your breakfast fix in, especially the pumpkin pie and maple walnut versions.

17. Keto Spinach and Artichoke Chicken

This juicy chicken has so many rich, delicious flavors happening at once that your taste buds will get a workout. You'll mix spinach, artichokes, garlic, cream cheese, mayo, and two types of cheese into a creamy paste, spread it all over the chicken and bake. Bubbly, cheesy goodness awaits after just 40 minutes, with little hands-on time.

18. Keto Grilled Chicken and Spinach Pizza

For a complete keto recipes list, we must include pizza, and this is the ultimate keto white pizza. It's got a crisp crust, white sauce, juicy chicken and fresh spinach. If you're following a keto diet, this pizza is a must-have for weekend nights.

19. Keto Zucchini Bread with Walnuts

This keto recipe is just as simple to make as a normal loaf of zucchini bread, with no crazy ingredients necessary. It's full of warm flavors, like cinnamon, ginger and nutmeg, plus it freezes well. Great to have for breakfast or as a snack.

20. Low-Carb Cheese Taco Shells

Anything tastes good when it's stuffed between these cheesy shells! These are so simple to make: it's just baked cheese! Stuff these with your favorite meats, veggies (bell peppers and onions are great here), taco fixings and, of course, more cheese!

21. Low-Carb Portabella Sliders

I love the low-carb take on traditional burgers: smaller patties nestled into portabella mushroom buns. These are simple to make and are made using a grill pan on the stove, so you can enjoy them year-round.

22. Secret Ingredient Easy Chocolate Mousse

I don't want to ruin the secret ingredient for this keto recipe, but suffice to say, it makes this mousse deliciously creamy! It's ready in just minutes, perfect for a last-minute dessert or late night chocolate craving.

23. Thai Beef Satay

Marinating the beef in this keto recipe infuses it with an impressive amount of flavor in just 15 minutes. While that happens, you can quickly mix together the peanut sauce and accompanying salad for this Asian-style weeknight meal.

24. The Ultimate Keto Buns

If you're missing traditional burger or sandwich buns, these keto-friendly buns will hit the spot. Using a stick blender, the dough is ready in seconds, and then they're finished off in the oven for fluffy buns that are just begging to be topped with your favorite meats and cheeses.

25. Vegan Alfredo

This rich and cheesy alfredo is not just keto and low-carb, it's vegan, too! You don't need to be vegan to appreciate how smooth and creamy this saucy favorite can be when made with almond milk, cauliflower and nutritional yeast. Keep it low-carb by serving over zucchini noodles.

Chapter 11

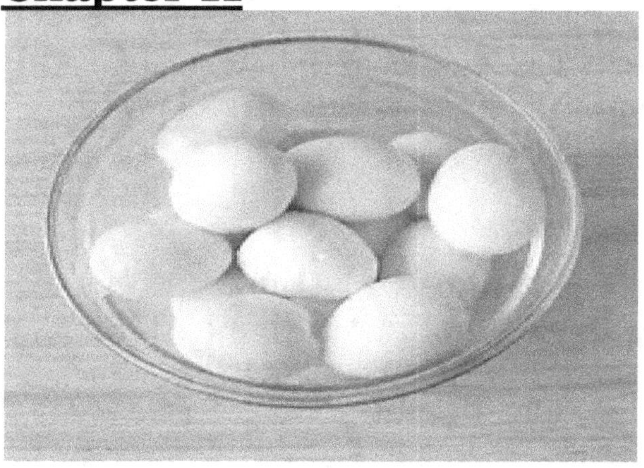

KETO RECIPES - ALL ABOUT EGGS

When on a Ketogenic diet (aka: Keto) you will learn real fast, that eggs are your new best friend. An easy, affordable way to get your fats and proteins in is by incorporating eggs into your daily diet. Sounds easy enough. Until you hit day 3 of course, and you're bored out of your mind of hard boiled eggs day after day. Something needs to change, and fast...or you're on a crash course to failing this meal plan. If you aren't ENJOYING the diet and lifestyle you're a part of, what's the point? So let us help you with some of the best Keto-friendly recipes to help you use up those eggs, in a way you WON'T get bored of them.

1. Keto McMuffin Sausage & Egg Breakfast Sandwich

When the egg becomes the bun... genius. The bun was just wasted space anyhow. With this one sandwich you're getting 32 grams of protein!

2. Avocado & Egg Fat Bombs

Another Keto staple food is avocados. High in fat (but the good kind!) they perfectly balance out a lot of ketogenic meal plans. This one recipe will make one of two things. Fat bombs (a term you will hear a lot with this diet plan), and deviled eggs!

3. Bacon & Egg Cups

YES there's a diet that you can eat a lot of BACON on. WOOP! This recipe makes muffin tins your best friend, when you line the cups with bacon, and crack a fresh egg into them. Bake the whole tray and you have a week's worth of snacks/meals!

4. Hollandaise Sauce

A simple way to add those healthy fats you need in your daily ketogenic diet, is a sauce made from eggs that you can use over eggs, meats or even some sliced avocado. It's incredibly rich, and will compliment so many dishes!

5. Avocado Bacon & Eggs

You need those avocados in your diet so why not make them the little boats to carry your eggs and bacon in. Don't get weirded out by the idea of a warm avocado, it's actually delicious! This easy recipe give you a breakfast or snack you know will give you all that energy boost you need.

6. Ham Hash Egg Cups

A perfect way to use up leftover ham, and it makes the most delicious hash for this egg recipe! This is also a recipe that you can make for yourself, but the whole family will love (kids tend to love that salty ham flavor).

7. Homemade Mayo

Okay, maybe not so much an "egg" recipe, but eggs are a big part of this recipe, and you will definitely get a lot of use out of it on a keto diet. If you've never made homemade mayo before, you are missing out! Give this one a try!

8. Egg Clouds

The first time I made these, I thought it must be rather unnecessary to mess with a common egg. Until I tried it. Talk about fluffy and amazing. You want to change up your egg game? THIS, is how.

9. Cobb Salad

A perfectly balanced keto meal that is nothing without those hard boiled eggs! Enjoy this incredible meal that will keep you full, and satisfied without being TOO heavy (like so many of the keto recipes out there tend to be). A full 43 grams of protein is packed in this single salad!

Chapter 12

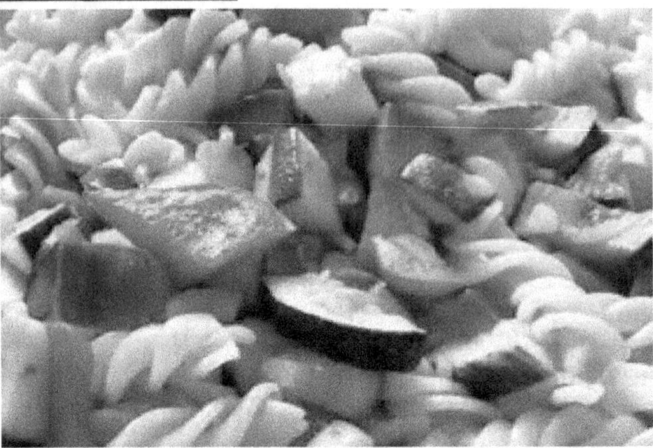

KETOGENIC PASTA RECIPES

Everybody loves pasta dishes. And the good news is, thanks to a few clever twists you can use to stay in ketosis, and still enjoy classic dishes like lasagna, spaghetti with meatballs, and chicken noodle soup.

You might find some new favorites in our list of keto pasta recipes – why not try the Cajun shrimp spaghetti, the Tuscan chicken pasta, the Asian garlic beef noodles or one of the many other recipes below.

TYPES OF KETO PASTA

How can you have pasta when you don't use wheat and other grains?

Don't worry, many of us have come up with other creative keto pasta by using ingredients such as Spaghetti squash, Zucchini, Cucumber, Eggplant (Aubergine), and Shirataki noodles.

While the exact texture and taste is slightly different from the pasta we're used to, these provide a new and healthier way of enjoying some old favorites.

Here are some tips to help you create "pasta" and "noodles" out of vegetables:

Spaghetti squash, cucumbers, and zucchini make great veggie noodles while eggplant is a tasty stand-in for lasagna sheets.

All you need is a spiralizer, a food processor with a shredding attachment, a kitchen grater, or even a potato peeler to create the noodles.

And to enjoy the noodles, you can add a classic sauce like tomato or bolognese, or you can try out a creative new one like the creamy avocado one.

Ketogenic Pasta Recipes

Ketogenic Pasta Recipes with Chicken

Creamy Tomato Basil Chicken Pasta

Ingredients: Chicken breasts, ghee or coconut oil, tomatoes, basil, coconut milk, garlic, salt, zucchini or spaghetti squash.

This is a quick and easy recipe which is ideal for a fast meal after a busy day. It can also be made quite cheaply so it is a great meal for students! The rich flavors of tomato and fragrant basil are so appealing, and make this dish taste amazing. If you don't have a spiralizer it doesn't matter, you can simply shred the zucchini in a food processor or using a grater.

Creamy Avocado "Pasta"

Ingredients: Zucchinis, chicken breast, Himalayan salt, black pepper, endive, asparagus spears, walnuts, parsley, avocado, full fat coconut milk, water, lemon juice, thyme.

Zucchini noodles make a delicious and healthy alternative to traditional pasta, and as they have a delicate flavor, are an ideal partner for rich sauces, or in this case a creamy avocado sauce. Spiralizers are easy to buy now, and are such fun to use a great way to get the kids involved in the kitchen too!

Chicken Noodle Soup

Ingredients: Chicken broth, chicken breast, avocado oil, celery, green onion, cilantro, zucchini, salt.

Chicken noodle soup is a favorite with so many of us, children included! This is a perfect recipe to encourage the kids to eat more veggies – they don't even think of the 'noodles' as vegetables! You can use a potato peeler to create thin strips, or treat yourself to a spiralizer and have fun making this.

Thai Chicken Pad

Ingredients: Chicken breast, green onion, broccoli florets, ginger, tamari sauce, garlic, cilantro, coconut oil, cucumber, salt.

Cucumber noodles are so easy to make you can slice them with a mandolin or just use a potato peeler to create the long flat strips. They add to the freshness of the flavor of this dish too. Remember that fresh ginger can be stored in the freezer and simply grated when needed, so you don't have any waste.

Pan-Fried Tuscan Chicken Pasta

Ingredients: Chicken breasts, egg, salt, black pepper, garlic powder, Italian seasoning, cherry tomatoes, basil leaves, olive oil or avocado oil, and zucchini.

Here is another quick recipe that is full of fresh flavors! Because the chicken is cooked quickly it keeps all its flavor, and doesn't dry out. Also basil and tomato is really a match made in heaven, so adding them to this pasta dish is a great idea. Basil is easy to grow in pots in the kitchen so you could have a source of freshness to add to soups, and sauces any time.

Ketogenic Pasta Recipes with Other Meats

Spaghetti Squash Bolognese

Ingredients: Spaghetti squash, ground or minced beef, onion, tomato, fresh basil, garlic, coconut oil, salt, and pepper.

Using spaghetti squash is a healthy alternative to traditional pasta, and can be eaten just the same way. This low carb recipe is a perfect way to introduce squash into your children's diet, and they could even learn to love it as much as they love pasta. By adding in the basil at the end of the cooking time it helps to retain the full freshness of the flavor.

Bacon-Basil Zucchini "Pasta"

Ingredients: Zucchini, salt, bacon grease, fresh basil, garlic cloves,and walnuts (optional).

Although this is technically a vegetable dish, it has been listed in this section because the recipe calls for bacon grease. You also have the option to add in crispy bacon bits too in order to make this keto pasta dish even more delicious. And if you choose to add in the walnuts, just be careful to keep stirring them to stop them from burning.

Lasagna with Eggplants

Ingredients: Ground pork, ground beef, onion, garlic, tomatoes, tomato paste, basil, fresh parsley, fresh oregano, fresh thyme, fennel seeds, eggs, coconut oil, salt, eggplant.

This is another versatile keto recipe swap the meats for your favorites or use zucchini instead of eggplant if you prefer. Fresh herbs add such amazing flavors to any dish that the resulting plate is appealing to the eye. Plus they give off wonderful aromas that will get your taste buds tingling before you even taste this lasagna.

Asian Garlic Beef Noodles

Ingredients: Onion, beef, avocado oil or coconut oil, tamari sauce, garlic, fresh ginger, cilantro, zucchini or shirataki noodles.

Ginger and garlic are the most common basic ingredients in Asian cuisine, and they make this dish taste so good! This keto noodle recipe is quite quick to make, giving you a speedy, tasty meal for unexpected dinner guests or after a busy day at work. The aromas from the beef will definitely make your mouth water! Try using a red onion instead for a gentler, slightly sweeter taste.

Ketogenic Pasta Recipes with Fish and Other Seafood

Garlic Roasted Shrimp With Zucchini Pasta

Ingredients: Shrimp, olive oil, ghee, garlic, lemon juice, lemon zest, salt, ground pepper, zucchini.

Shrimp is a fabulous ingredient to serve with keto pasta as it gives a real diversity if texture to the dish. It also gives you a lighter option than using beef, and could even be spiced up a bit if you like with the addition of some chili flakes. And of course we all know how well lemon goes with fish.

Zucchini Noodles with Scallops & Bacon

Ingredients: Bay scallops, bacon, zucchini, garlic powder, green onions, lemon juice, sea salt, and black pepper.

What an impressive dish this is! The tiny scallops and meaty bacon pieces make this a meal to impress for a dinner party or celebration. Because the zucchini noodles do not have a strong flavor, don't be tempted to skimp on the seasoning as they take on stronger flavors really well. If you can't find the tiny scallops then use large ones, and slice them through the middle.

Zucchini Pasta with Spicy Shrimp Marinara

Ingredients: Zucchinis, shrimp, salt, smoked paprika, cooking fat of choice, diced tomatoes, olive oil, garlic, Italian seasoning, fresh basil, crushed red pepper.

The smoked paprika in this recipe helps give you a delicious smokey flavor that goes well with the shrimp. If you can't find smoked paprika, then regular paprika also works well. To prepare the zucchini you can use a mandolin, a shredder setting on a food processor or why not try investing in a spiralizer.

Cajun Shrimp Spaghetti

Ingredients: Shrimp, zucchini, onion, coconut milk, stock, arrowroot starch, cajun seasoning, garlic powder, black pepper, and olive oil.

Shrimp has long been an ingredient associated with Cajun cuisine, and this recipe is no different. The shrimp can easily handle the Cajun seasoning. The shrimp also gives you a lovely meaty texture which goes so well with the softer texture of the zucchini. If you prefer, you could use red onion to add a different color, and a gentler flavor, but because of the spice the white onion tastes great.

Zoodles With Sardines, Tomatoes & Capers

Ingredients: Sardines packed in olive oil, extra virgin olive oil, garlic, ripe tomatoes, capers, zucchini noodles, salt, pepper, parsley.

Sardines are a great source of omega-3, making them a great addition for increasing the health benefits of your food. They have quite a strong flavor which is great when teamed with the zoodles and capers, giving a Mediterranean-type taste. This meal is gluten, dairy and egg-free, so is a perfect option for guests or family members who have health difficulties.

Garlic Oregano Olive Tapenade

Ingredients: Olives, oregano leaves, garlic, extra virgin olive oil, zucchini, and sardines.

This is a quick and easy recipe for a tapenade that is served here with sardines. But if you don't like sardines, you can also use grilled chicken or fish instead. In our house olive tapenade has also been served as a dip for veggie crudities. The oregano provides a lovely fresh flavor, and the olives add the richness. This is a good way to introduce olives to your diet if you have never tried them before.

Vegetarian Ketogenic Pasta Recipes

Zucchini Pasta Pesto

Ingredients: Zucchini, roasted garlic walnut pesto, cherry tomatoes, fresh basil, sea salt.

Sometimes a simple dish like this is just what we need – packed with fresh flavors, and so tasty it will keep you coming back! Pesto makes a great addition to a pasta dish, and this recipe is a great way to use up home-grown basil and tomatoes. This makes a great meal on its own or you could add some protein by including chicken or shrimp.

Coconut Oil Baked Spaghetti Squash

Ingredients: Spaghetti squash, and coconut oil.

This is a basic recipe for cooking spaghetti squash to which you can add protein and sauce of your choice. Spaghetti squash can also be micro-waved, but the oven-cooked way tastes better. It is also a great way to introduce the kids to eating healthier options than traditional pasta.

Zucchini Pasta With Avocado Cream Sauce

Ingredients: Zucchini, avocado, cucumber, lemon juice, garlic, coconut milk, basil, salt, pepper, cherry tomatoes.

This dish makes a lovely side dish to be served on summer evenings. It's full of fresh flavors, and can be used along with grilled chicken or fish. The colors are so appealing, thanks to the basil and tomatoes, and the taste is zingy because of the lemon juice. The zucchini can be cut with a spiralizer or mandolin.

Zucchini "Pasta" with Coriander and Cashew Pesto (Contains Dairy)

Ingredients: Coriander, garlic, red long chili, raw cashews, Parmesan cheese, macadamia oil, sea salt flakes, and black pepper.

Pesto can always be associated with fresh flavors, and this pasta dish is a light a fragrant option for a summery dinner. This is a vegetarian dish, but could also be served with pulled pork or chicken for extra protein. If you don't like chili, then simply leave it out and enjoy the natural herby freshness from the coriander.

Guacamole Pasta

Ingredients: Zucchinis, garlic, baby spinach, lime juice, olive oil, avocados, sea salt, grape tomatoes, and jalapeño (optional).

This recipe is so quick and easy to make and the result is a light and summery meal that is full of flavors and textures. The creaminess of the avocado and garlic guacamole is a perfect partner to the zucchini noodles. You can also use the guac as a dip with vegetable crudities for a party or celebration.

Zucchini Noodles

Ingredients: Tomato sauce, coconut milk, onion powder, garlic powder, dried basil, red pepper flakes, salt, black pepper, olive oil, zucchini, avocado oil, Prosciutto and goat cheese (optional).

Sometimes you just have to have pasta with sauce. This keto pasta recipe gives you a rich and creamy tomato sauce which is delicious on its own. If you want some protein as well, you can drop it in for a more filling meal.

Live Pasta with Agretti and Lemon

Ingredients: Extra virgin olive oil, garlic cloves, lemon juice, lemon zest, agretti, and zucchini.

Agretti is a vegetable specific to Italy and is not that easy to find, although it is well worth searching it out. If you can't find it you can substitute spinach. Some folks prefer their zucchini noodles cooked to make them softer. If this is you then simply cook them for a couple of minutes. But be careful not to move them around too much or they will break up.

Easy Spaghetti with Tomato Sauce

Ingredients: Onion, tomatoes, Italian seasoning, bell pepper, zucchini, garlic, basil, olive oil, salt, pepper, cucumber noodles or shirataki noodles.

Have you ever been in the position of having to rustle up a quick lunch when someone drops in unexpectedly? Especially challenging if the guest is vegetarian? Well, keep this recipe filed away and it provides you with a light meal that makes the most of fresh flavors and ingredients that most of us keep regularly. The Italian seasoning and basil give this dish a true flavor of the Mediterranean! If you have shirataki noodles handy, then feel free to use those here or else use a cucumber for a nice refreshing effect.

BREAKFAST

Breakfast is a pivotal meal for staying in ketosis. You've been asleep, which is an automatic fast so your body is most likely in ketosis already, especially if you were eating low carb the day before. This is a prime opportunity to load up on some more fat for fuel for the day. But breakfast can also be a chaotic time of day for you as you try to find Easy low carb recipes for your Ketogenic diet menu. Kids, pets, or forgetting to do laundry the day before are all things that can make the early hours of the day a race against the clock.

So with our two easy low carb recipes for your Ketogenic diet menu breakfast, we're going to give you one that takes less preparation, and one that's a bit more intricate.

Recipe 1. QUICK BREAKFAST

If you're REALLY in a hurry, we suggest going with a Bulletproof Coffee. Caffeine, calories, and FAT, and the best part is that you can sip it on your way to work.

Recipe in its simplest form (there are other variations that spice it up):

1 to 2 tablespoons of unsalted (preferably organic) butter.

1 tablespoon of MCT Oil (If you do not currently own MCT Oil, we would suggest purchasing some. BUT you can substitute coconut oil for the time being. If you do this, you should double the serving (2 tablespoons).

1 to 2 cups of black coffee (preferably organic). No fufu sugar bomb coffee. Legit black jet fuel.

QUICKY RECIPE:

Piggy Avo Scramble

Ingredients:

Two Eggs

One Avocado

2 Slices of bacon

Instructions: Fry slices of bacon in frying pan and remove.

Scramble two eggs in bowl and pour into pan with bacon grease.

While eggs cook, chop bacon and avocado into small pieces.

Once eggs are near completion, add bacon and avocado to mix and finish.

Recipe 2. Keto Omelet

Ingredients:

One serving ground pork sausage

4 eggs

1 cup shredded cheddar cheese

1 cup spinach

½ chopped avocado

1 tablespoon olive oil

Toppings (optional): 1 tablespoon sour cream and 1 teaspoon Tabasco hot sauce

Instructions: Cook sausage until done. Once done, remove from pan.

Place Olive Oil in pan.

Scramble eggs in bowl and add to pan after removing sausage.

Once bottom of eggs have started to solidify, add sausage, cheese, and vegetables to one half of the eggs. (Remember, you're going to fold this over!)

Once eggs are cooked enough, fold empty side of eggs over on top of side with fillings (like a taco).

Let the folded egg cook on lowered heat until inside of omelet is completely cooked. Be sure to not burn the outsides of the omelet!

Once cooked thoroughly, remove omelet, top with sour cream and hot sauce and enjoy!

LUNCH

By this time of the day, the hunger is setting in. You need to nail this meal to have the energy to make it through the rest of the day, plus an afternoon workout (if you exercise after work). Easy low carb recipes for your Ketogenic diet menu will keep you from wondering off to the vending machine during the dreaded two o'clock drag that inevitably happens.

We also realize that you have coworkers, and they sometimes pressure you into going out to lunch. We're going to prepare you for that too!

Recipe 1. Keto Cowboy Burgers

Ingredients:

2 tablespoons olive oil

1 egg

1 pound 70%/30% ground beef

1 tablespoon season salt

4 slices bacon

1 yellow onion

1 cup sliced jalapeños

2 slices pepper jack cheese

Primal Kitchen Chipotle Mayo

PREPERATION TO GO!

Add two tablespoons of olive oil to cast iron skillet (or frying pan), and bring to medium heat.

In medium mixing bowl, add hamburger and season salt. Break egg into hamburger and mix thoroughly.

Sculpt hamburger mix into two large patties and place into pan.

Fry on both sides, keeping mind to turn the burgers often to avoid overdoing one side.

Cut slit in center of burger with spatula and press. If fluid from burger is clear, it is done. If it runs red, it still needs to cook longer.

Before removing patties, place slices of cheese on top of patties, and slightly melt them onto burgers.

While patties are cooking, slice onion and mix them with the jalapeños.

Once patties are removed, add onion/jalapeño mix into the pan, and let them caramelize in the grease.

TRAVEL PREP

In a travel container place patties in first, and then top with caramelized vegetables. Put mayo into separate container.

When ready to eat, put mayo on both patties after reheating.

Recipe 2. Quick Keto Salad

Ingredients:

Meat Options: Chicken or Steak

If chicken: Place chicken breasts in crockpot and cook on low overnight to shred meat for salad the next day.

Ingredients: 4 chicken breasts, 2 cups of stock, and sprinkle dry ranch dressing over the top of the chicken. Shred apart with forks!

If steak: Season and cook two ribeye steaks on grill to preferred doneness and cut into bite sized pieces.

1 tablespoon olive oil

1 serving ranch dressing

1/2 cup shredded cheese (preferably cheddar)

2 cups mixed greens

Mix meat with greens in travel container

Keep oil, dressing, and cheese separate until you're ready to eat your salad! (If you put the dressing on beforehand, it will cause the greens to wilt and produce a gross texture).

Once you're ready to eat, put tablespoon olive oil, serving of ranch, and cheese on top of your salad and enjoy!

DINNER

You'll be able to be most creative with your Ketogenic diet menu at dinner time. This is the time where you're chilling out, and able to focus on a large scale meal that will meet your keto needs, while also bringing some adventure to your eating day.

But for the sake of versatility, we'll be providing you with two easy low carb recipes; one being more intricate, the other being a crockpot recipe you can throw in at the start of the day, and just throw on a plate when you get home from a busy day.

Recipe 1. Slow Cooker Crockpot Pork with Greens

Ingredients:

One pork roast

One packet Au Jus seasoning

One packet of ranch dressing seasoning

One stick of unsalted butter

5 cups collard greens

Instructions: Place pork roast in crockpot and spread greens over the roast and throughout the crock.

Sprinkle Au Jus and Ranch evenly across roast and greens.

Place stick of butter on top of the roast in the center.

Cook on medium to low (depending on the crockpot) for 6 to 8 hours.

All you need to do when you get home is scoop it out onto your plate and enjoy!

RECIPE 2. CHICKEN ZOODLE SPAGHETTI

Ingredients:

One 12.5 oz can of canned chicken

¼ block of velveeta cheese cubed into small pieces

3 to 4 medium sized zucchini

One tablespoon of oil

One can of rotel

You'll need to cut the zucchini into zoodles.

Instructions: Once you've spiralized your zucchini, you'll need to cook it down for five to ten minutes on medium heat in a frying pan, with one tablespoon of olive oil, adding some water while it cooks to ensure the zoodles retain moisture.

As your zoodles cook, add the velveeta and begin melting it down.

Once the cheese is melted down, add the rotel and can chicken.

Cook for another five minutes to heat mixture completely through.

Scoop onto plate, and enjoy!

These easy low carb recipes for your Ketogenic diet menu will make life a lot easier, while keeping your diet interesting. There's no reason why you can't stay enthusiastic about your meal while also maintaining your principles you just have to be creative.

Whether you're a stay at home parent, or someone working 60+ hours a week at an office, you can stick to your Ketogenic diet! It just take knowledge paired with preparation, which gives birth to execution.

Keto Meal 1: Breakfast Buns

These buns are amazing, and really good for anyone who misses bread, burger buns or something to scoop up sauces! They're delicious with some butter or ghee on each half, topped with 2 slices of Parma ham.

Ingredients:

1.5 cups Macadamia nuts, unsalted

3 Eggs, organic

1 tsp Cider Vinegar

1/4 cup coconut milk (Tetra Pak)

60g + 12 tbsp Butter (1 tbsp for each half)

1/3 cup Almond flour

1/3 cup Coconut flour

1 tsp Bicarbonate of Soda (Baking Soda)

1 tsp Rock Salt pink

Instructions: Preheat the oven to 160C/325F.

Grind the macadamia nuts to a coarse flour in a strong food processor.

Add eggs, vinegar, milk and butter. Process until you have a smooth paste.

Put all the dry ingredients into a bowl and stir well. Add wet to dry and mix until you have a wet dough.

Form 6 buns and bake for 25 minutes. Spread 1 tbsp of butter onto each half. Eat on the same day or freeze.

Keto Meal 2: Almond Coconut Pancakes

Ingredients:

1 tsp ground Cinnamon

1/2 cup desiccated Coconut

1 1/2 cup ground blanched Almonds

1/2 tsp Baking soda/ Bicarbonate of soda

1/4 tsp Sea Salt

1 cup Coconut milk canned

3 large Eggs organic or free range

2 tbsp (solid) Coconut oil

Cooking Instructions

Sift dry ingredients and mix together.

Instructions: In a separate bowl, whisk coconut milk and eggs together.

Add dry ingredients and mix thoroughly.

Heat coconut oil in a pan, pour in batter and cook for 2 to 3 minutes per side.

Keto Meal 3: Rainbow Salad

Ingredients:

2 cups chopped Butterhead Lettuce

1 small young Carrot, grated

4 sticks Celery, sliced

8 tbsp grated Celeriac, raw

2 tbsp Shelled Hemp Seeds

4 tsp Pumpkin Seeds

12 tbsp raw Alfalfa sprouts

240g Smoked or Grilled Trout

1/2 cup Avocado oil

2 tsp Cider Vinegar

2 tsp Mustard Dijon smooth

Salt and Black Pepper to taste

80g Cheese, e.g. Gruyere

Instructions: Toss the vegetables, hemp/pumpkin seeds, sprouts, and trout into a bowl and mix with the butterhead leaves.

Mix the avocado oil, apple cider vinegar, mustard and seasoning, and pour over the salad. Grate some fresh Gruyère over it. This one really pops with color.

Keto Meal 4: Bacon Brussels Sprouts

Ingredients:

3 tbsp Coconut oil

5 Bacon rashers, diced

1 clove Garlic, crushed

500g Brussels sprouts, shredded

1 Leek, thinly sliced

Salt and Black Pepper

3/4 cup Chicken Stock, homemade

Instructions: Cook the bacon in coconut oil in a large frying pan over medium heat until crisp.

Remove the bacon from the pan and set aside. Add the shredded Brussels sprouts, leek and garlic to the pan and sauté in the remaining oil for 5 minutes.

Add the chicken broth, salt and pepper. Cover and steam for 5-10 minutes. Mix in the bacon.

Keto Meal 5: Liver Mousse

One of my missions is to get my clients to incorporate more fat-vitamin-rich, hormone-nourishing organ meat into their diet! I know…it's not an easy goal. This recipe is inspired by Jasmine and Melissa Hemsley.

Ingredients:

200g organic Chicken liver, raw

1/2 Apple

100g Butter, at room temperature

2 organic Eggs

1/2 Small Onion

1/2 tsp ground Allspice

1 tsp Rock Salt and 1/2 tsp Black Pepper

Instructions: Preheat the oven to 130C/250F.

Put all ingredients into a strong blender and pulse until you have a smooth paste.

Fill into a muffin tin and bake for 20-25 minutes.

YOUR KETO RECIPES FOR WEIGHT LOSS

The Keto Friendly Pancakes

We've said no refined carbs so your first thought may have been that pancakes are out of the question. That's where you're wrong. The trick is to work around this grain-free, carb-free world to create your favorite breakfast.

Rather than pancakes, I have some pancake muffins for you. You get the best of both worlds with this recipe!

Ingredients:

12 cup yoghurt—whole milk and plain

2 tbsp coconut oil or unsalted butter, melted

1 tsp vanilla extract

¼ tsp apple cider vinegar

1 ¾ cup almond flour

½ tsp baking soda

1 tsp salt

3 eggs

Instructions:

1. Place muffin cups in your 6-12 space tray.

2. Preheat oven to 350 degrees.

3. Blend your yoghurt, oil, vinegar, extract and any sweetener you have together. Add the flour, salt, and baking soda. Blend until combined.

4. Now add in the eggs and blend again. Pop it on a high setting and blend for about 30 seconds until the eggs just mix in to create your batter.

5. Now add in all your other ingredients and stir by hand.

6. Place the batter into your muffin liners. Add some chopped walnuts or almonds on top if you wish.

7. Bake for around 15-20 minutes. To test if they're done, stick a knife or skewer into the middle and see if it comes out clean. If not, then the muffins need to go back in for a little longer.

You can add in some sweetener if you find you need it in your muffins. Opt for a natural sweetener like Stevia if you're going to use it. You can also add some nuts and seeds into the mix for that little extra bite. Poppy seeds work really well.

Some keto recipes do add some blueberries and raspberries to them. While we say no fruits allowed, there are some fruits that work out lower in carbs. You can create muffins with 4.5g net carbs by adding some fruits.

Allow them to cool before you serve/eat.

Poppy Seed Muffins

If you're not the biggest fan of the pancake muffins, why not try these poppy seed muffins instead? These muffins work great when served with cream cheese to add a little extra fat to your diet. See here some awesome muffin pan.

Ingredients:

¾ cup almond flour

¼ cup flaxseed meal

1/3 cup natural sweetener like Erythritol

1 tsp baking powder

¼ cup unsalted butter

¼ cup double cream

2 tbsp poppy seeds

3 eggs

3 tbsp lemon juice

1 tsp vanilla extract

Natural sweetener to taste

Instructions:

1. Preheat the oven to 350°.

2. Combine the flour, flaxseed, erythritol, and seeds.

3. Melt the butter. Stir it into the flour with the cream and eggs. Create a smooth batter.

4. Add the rest of the ingredients.

5. Place 12 cupcake moulds onto a baking tray. Pour the mixture evenly over them. Silicone moulds are great for keeping the regular cost down.

6. Bake for around 20 minutes, until brown. You can also do the skewer test mentioned above.

7. Allow to cool before serving

This mixture of ingredients will give you just 1.5g net carbs per muffin. They can be quite small, but will help to curb some of that sweet tooth. The best part is you feel like you're being naughty without actually piling on the pounds.

Try serving by cutting in half and placing butter or cream cheese in between the halves. They can make a great breakfast or snack.

Pizza Breakfast Frittata

Have you ever just wanted pizza for breakfast? Of course, you have, but that's not allowed on the keto diet, is it? Well, here's a slight variation to keep you happy throughout the week.

Ingredients:

12 eggs

9 oz spinach ripped into smaller pieces

1 oz pepperoni

1 tsp garlic, minced

5 oz mozzarella cheese

½ cup ricotta cheese

4 tbsp oil

¼ tsp nutmeg

Seasoning to taste

Instructions:

1. Preheat the oven to 375°.

2. Mix the eggs, spices and oil together.

3. Add in the cheese and spinach.

4. Add to a skillet, sprinkle with some extra mozzarella cheese on top.

5. Add the pepperoni to make it look like a pizza.

6. Place in the oven and bake for 30 minutes.

Serve with your favorite fatty dressings.

This isn't going to be your quick morning breakfast, but it is great for getting everyone to sit together on the weekend.

Mock McGriddle Loaf

Who said a loaf was going to be completely off the list? You can always make your own keto friendly options, and there are plenty of ideas out there. This is just one of the best ones available.

The best part about this keto recipe is that you can make it the night or even the day before. It keeps in the fridge for a few days, so you have a great quick breakfast idea.

Ingredients:

1 cup almond flour

¼ cup flaxseed

1lb sausage

10 eggs

4 oz cheese—cheddar or something similar

6 tbsp maple syrup

4 tbsp butter

½ tsp onion powder

½ tsp garlic powder

¼ tsp sage

Seasoning to taste

Instructions:

1. Pre-heat the oven to 350°.

2. Add the sausage to a pan on the stove. Break up and cook until brown.

3. Place all the dry ingredients into a bowl. Combine and add the wet ingredients, except 2 tbsp maple syrup.

4. Add the sausage into the mixture.

5. Place parchment paper into a casserole dish, and add the mixture in.

6. Drizzle the remaining syrup over.

7. Bake for around 50 minutes, until completely cooked through.

8. Remove and allow to cool.

Try serving with some syrup or ketchup. It's perfect for that Sunday morning treat.

Burger buns may not be allowed on the keto diet, but that doesn't mean you can't opt for a burger for your lunch. This burger with a twist is a great alternate option.

I've already mentioned using spinach leaves for the bun, but what about using two burgers for the bun instead? They have plenty of fat, especially if you fry them in olive oil. You can add all the toppings you want and finish it off with a side salad or some fries—again, with a slight twist.

Ingredients:

800g minced beef

8 rashers of bacon, chopped

¼ cup cheese, something like cheddar

2 tbsp chives, chopped

Slices of onion

2 tsp garlic, minced

Salt and Pepper to taste

Soy sauce/Worcestershire sauce to taste

Instructions:

1. Start by frying your bacon in a pan with some oil. Season as you like.

2. Once fully cooked, remove the bacon and place on some paper towels to soak up the oils.

3. Now mix your beef with all the ingredients, except the cheese, in a mixing bowl.

4. Create patties with your hands. You should be able to get 8-10 patties.

5. Fry each of the patties in your oil. You should be able to cook at least two at once.

6. Flip the burgers and cook until they are made just the way you like.

You can also add other toppings that you like. Try some tomatoes, pickles, and more! You could spice things up by adding some extra flavors to your beef burgers. You could also add some jalapenos or chili if you like a kick.

If you want something a little lighter on the stomach, consider some turkey mince or pork mince instead.

To serve, place one patty on the plate, and then top with some cheese, extra bacon and all the vegetables you want.

Top with the second Pattie. Top with all the fatty dressing you could want.

French Fry Substitute

Did you think reading all this that you couldn't have fries again? I'm happy to tell you that fries are definitely allowed.

However, these won't be the fries that you know best. You'll need to make substitutes with Daikon radish. I'd never heard of this before learning about the keto diet, but I'm glad I did. You can also make fries out of other root vegetables, like butternut squash and parsnips.

You may need to go to an Asian butcher to find a Daikon radish because this is the region the vegetable comes from. It's used in plenty of Asian dishes.

The best thing about the fries is that they couldn't be easier to make. You can then top them with your favorites like bacon and cheese, and opt for sauces like ketchup and ranch dressing.

Ingredients:

1 daikon radish, sliced into fries

¼ cup coconut oil

Pinch of sea salt

Spices to taste

Instructions:

1. Preheat the oven to 475°.

2. Place the radish strips into a bag.

3. Pour in the melted coconut oil, salt, and spices. Tie up the bag, and shake until the radish strips are completely coated.

4. Spread the strips on the tray.

5. Bake for about 15 minutes, flip, and then bake for another 15 minutes.

6. Remove and allow to cool before serving.

The best length for these fries will be around 3", and you'll want them about a 1/2" thick. Make sure you wash the radish to get rid of the starch on it. Baking times will depend on the thickness, so keep an eye on your fries while they're cooking. If they look finished, they probably are.

Serve them on the side of your burger.

Cauliflower Grilled Cheese

It's not just fries and pizza that are still allowed when you find a twist. You can also opt for a grilled cheese sandwich. The different is you're substituting the bread for cauliflower crust.

Cauliflower has become a great substitute for the likes of pasta and bread dishes. Cauliflower crust can also be used for pizza bases, which you can top with absolutely anything you want.

To get started with this recipe, you need to create your cauliflower crust for the bread, and you can use this for your burger if you really want a pun for the patties.

Start by grating your cauliflower, so it looks like cauliflower rice. Put it all in a bowl and squeeze out as much moisture as possible. This helps to pack everything

together to make your bread slices. Make the cauliflower
into patties and then pop onto a baking tray. Just put in
the oven on a medium heat for around 15 minutes.
They'll be ready to go!

Yes, your bread substitute is really that easy. Of course, if
you want a pizza base, you turn the cauliflower into a
larger base. And get creative with shapes. Your
imagination is your limit.

Grilled Cheese

Ingredients:

4 slices of cauliflower crust

The amount of cheese you want and the type of cheese
you would prefer is up to you.

Instructions:

1. Heat a skillet over medium heat with a bit of oil.

2. Add one slice of cauliflower crust.

3. Top with your cheese and optionally other ingredients.

4. Add the top slice.

5. Cook until the cheese is melting out of the sides.
Remember to flip to prevent one side burning!

This is a super simple lunch. You can add in all the extras
that you would like. Some love cheese and tomato
sandwiches, while others prefer to throw in some onion.
There are some who just love grilled cheese on its own,
with plenty of cheese.

You can also season your sandwich to taste. And don't
forget a dip for it on the side.

To get the golden look, butter the side of the cauliflower crust that is at the base of your pan.

Chicken & Mushroom Celery Root Pasta

This is a great low-carb pasta option using the celery root as a pasta substitute. It looks and tastes very much like chicken noodle soup. Over time, you'll barely even realise that you've not had noodles, pasta or rice in a while.

Ingredients:

2 celery roots

1 tbsp ghee

½ tsp salt

Ingredients for sauce:

1 ¾ cups of water

½ cup of cashew nuts

1 tbsp ghee

1 tbsp lemon juice

Garlic and onion powder, and salt

Ingredients for the meat and vegetables

3 cups of chopped mushrooms

2-4 chicken breasts, skinless

2 tbsp ghee

Garlic and onion powder, and salt

¼ cup of water

Instructions:

Start with the sauce and noodles

1. Peel your celery root and spiralize them. Sprinkle with salt.

2. Heat on a medium pan and place the spiralized celery in it. Add the ghee.

3. Saute until they are easily halved.

4. Blend all the ingredients for the sauce and then pour over the noodles. Simmer while partially covered on a low heat. Leave for about 20 minutes, while you work on the other part.

Mushrooms and chicken:

1. Saute the mushrooms over a medium heat.

2. Add the ghee and salt.

3. Leave until tender.

4. In another pan add ghee.

5. Sprinkle your chicken with the seasoning on both sides and then cook for a minute on both sides.

6. Add the water and place a lid over the pan with a slight crack.

7. Reduce the heat and cook for about 20 minutes.

8. Leave to cool and cut the chicken up into pieces.

9. Add the chicken and mushrooms to the noodles.

10. Mix together and serve with seasoning to taste.

The root vegetables mix in with the sauce, making anyone believe they're really eating pasta.

Chicken Tikka Masala

Curries are popular dishes, especially a tikka masala. The great news is that you can still have one on the keto diet. You just need to substitute your rice for some cauliflower rice, and that is really simple and delicious to make.

The best way to cook this is with a slow cooker. Get everything in the pot, and leave it to do the hard work for you. It's a great way to set something for dinner and leave it until after work. You can make it in the oven if you wish.

Ingredients:

1 1/2lbs chicken thighs, leave the skin on and bone in

1lb chicken thighs without the skin and bone

2 tbsp olive oil

2 tsp onion powder

1 in ginger root, grated

3 garlic cloves, minced

Mixture of tomato paste, garam masala, smoke paprika, and salt

10 oz can of tomatoes, diced

1 cup coconut milk

1 cup double cream

Guar gum and cilantro to taste

Instructions:

1. De-bone your chicken and chop all the chicken into pieces. Keep the skin on them.

2. Add all the chicken into the slow cooker, and grate the ginger over the top.

3. Add everything up to, (but not including) the coconut milk into the slow cooker. Mix everything together.

4. Add half the coconut milk.

5. Cook for 3 hours on high or 6 hours on low.

6. Once cooked, add the rest of the ingredients and mix.

Serve your curry over your cauliflower rice. Simple grate some cauliflower, and place in a microwaveable bowl. Pop in the microwave for about a minute, and then place on your plate as a bed for the curry. You'll barely tell the difference!

Instead of the rice, you can also create a bed of mixed vegetables for your curry.

Chicken and Broccoli Stuffed Courgettes

Another great dinner option is stuffed courgettes. You can add all the vegetables and meat that you want, but this recipe will use broccoli and chicken.

Ingredients:

2 courgettes, hallowed out with 1in left near the skin

2 tbsp butter

3 oz cheese, shredded

6 oz chicken, shredded

1 cup broccoli

2 tbsp sour cream

1 stalk of green onion

Seasoning to taste

Instructions:

1. Preheat oven to 400°.

2. Melt your butter, and pour into the hallowed courgette. Season and place in the oven.

3. Cook the courgettes while following the rest of the steps.

4. Cut up your broccoli, and then combine it with the chicken and sour cream in a bowl. Season well.

5. Once the courgette is cooked (should take 20 minutes) take it out of the oven, and fill with the chicken.

6. Sprinkle with cheese.

7. Place back in the oven for about 10 minutes, until the cheese is melted.

8. Garnish with your green onion.

Cauliflower and Jalapeno Cheese

Now it's time to give your cauliflower cheese a bit of a spicy twist. This is one of those great dishes that works with everything, and is even a dinner by itself. You can make it a side dish for Thanksgiving or opt for it as a main meal packed with vegetables, and even throw in some bacon.

Consider adding some spiralised veggies, so it feels like you're getting some pasta in your dish. It'll feel like a twist on mac 'n' cheese.

Ingredients for the puree:

1 cauliflower head

2 tbsp double cream

1 tbsp butter

¼ cup cheese grated

1 tbsp jalapenos, chopped

¼ tsp garlic powder

Seasoning to taste

Ingredients for the cheese:

6 oz cream cheese

½ cup cheese, shredded

¼ cup of salsa

Ingredients for the topping:

¾ cup Colby jack cheese grated

¼ cup jalapenos, sliced

Insturctions:

Start with the puree:

1. Preheat the oven at 375°.

2. Break the cauliflower into medium sized pieces. Pop in the microwave with the cream and butter and cook for

10 minutes. Coat with the melted cream and butter, and put in the microwave for another 6minutes.

3. Remove and place in a blender with the rest of the ingredients. Blend until pureed.

Cream Cheese

1. Place the cream cheese in a bowl, and microwave for 30 seconds.

2. Add the cheese and salsa, mixing completely.

Casserole

1. Spread the puree across a casserole dish.

2. Spread the cream cheese over the top.

3. Layer with your toppings.

4. Bake for 20 minutes.

If you're going to add the vegetables or bacon, do this with the cream cheese layer. You can also serve with crumbled bacon over the top.

Keto Friendly Sushi

Sushi is a delicious dish, but what do you do when it comes to all that rice? How do you get around it all? Well, you can. Here is a look at a keto friendly recipe for sushi to try out when you have some time.

Do bear in mind that sushi can take some time to make.

The trick with the rice is to find a substitute, and we've already looked at cauliflower rice. Avoid over grating your cauliflower. You don't want it so fine that it is a fine powder for this dish. It still needs to have a rice texture. You will also need to add some cream cheese to the cauliflower to work for this rice substitute. Otherwise you'll just get the cauliflower everywhere.

It's worth having a bamboo roller to make your sushi. This will help to keep everything packed together as you go. If you don't have one, use some parchment paper to help with the roll.

Ingredients:

16 oz cauliflower

6 oz softened cream cheese

2 tbsp rice vinegar

5 nori sheets

1 tbsp soy sauce

1 mini cucumber

2 avocados

5 oz of seafood of your choice

Instructions:

1. Grate the cauliflower.

2. Slice the ends of your cucumber off, and then tip it so it's upright. Slice in half and discard the middle of both. Slice into strips, and set to one side.

3. Add your cauliflower into a very hot pan. Season with soy sauce as it cooks.

4. Add the cauliflower to a bowl. Mix in the cream cheese and vinegar. Set in the fridge to cool down.

5. Once the rice is cooled, slice your avocado into small strips, and remove the shell.

6. Place a nori sheet onto your bamboo roller. Spread on the rice, leaving about 3/4in at the top.

7. Place your fillers layering just the way you want.

8. Roll the sushi with your bamboo roller. This will take some practice to get right.

Serve with some wasabi and pickled ginger. You'll feel like you're in a Japanese restaurant, enjoying a local dish.

Chocolate and Coconut Bars

When you feel like a snack, sometimes you just want to reach for the chocolate. This is something that you can do on the keto diet, but you need just the right type of recipe. Well, I've got you covered when it comes to your snacking needs. This tastes just like a Bounty bar. You can make it as long or short as you want, and even cut it into bite-sized chunks for easy snacking on the go.

A coconut is a great option for a snack on the keto diet because it's so fatty. This is just what you need, right! But, doesn't chocolate have the sugar and carbs? Well, there's a slight secret to this, and you'll see once you look at the ingredients.

Ingredients:

1 cup unsweetened coconut, desiccated

1 packet natural sweetener like stevia

1 tsp vanilla extract

1/3 cup coconut cream

4 tbsp coconut oil/cocoa butter

2 tbsp cocoa powder, unsweetened

Instructions:

1. Mix the coconut, cream, extract, and stevia together. Blend with a spoon.

2. Line a cookie sheet with parchment paper and place the coconut mixture on it.

3. Shape into a rectangle about 1in thick.

4. Freeze for two hours. It will be solid.

5. While this happens, you can melt your coconut oil/cocoa butter (whichever you choose) in a sauce pan.

6. Add the powder, and some stevia and extract the oil. Mix and heat for 2 minutes.

7. Allow to cool until at room temperature.

8. Remove the coconut from the freezer, and cut into bars.

9. Dip the bars into the cocoa mixture, coating all sides evenly.

10. Place onto the cookie sheet, and put into the fridge to cool completely.

11. Allow to remain in the fridge to keep the solid consistency when it comes to eating them.

If you want them softer, allow reaching room temperature.

There, you have your Bounty snacks. But what about dessert? It's time to try out these last two keto recipes for weight loss.

Chocolate Mug Cake

You should know by now that just because we say carbs and sugar are banned that it doesn't mean you can't find ways around things. Yes, you really still can have a cake. The best thing about it is that it's real simple to make. You don't need your oven!

This will make one serving so you can benefit from a quick dessert just for you. You could substitute the almond flour for protein powder if you want. It doesn't quite give the right consistency and texture, but have a play around with it and test it out.

Ingredients:

1 egg

2 tbsp butter

2 tbsp almond butter/protein powder

2 tbsp cocoa powder, unsweetened

1 ½ tbsp Splenda

2 tsp coconut flour

¼ tsp vanilla extract

½ tsp baking powder

Insturctions:

1. Get your mug and put your butter into it.

2. Microwave for about 25 seconds until hot and melted. Add the sweetener.

3. Add the cocoa powder, coconut and almond flours, extract, baking powder, and egg.

4. Mix until completely combined.

5. You'll need to make sure there are no lumps for this to turn out just right.

6. Microwave for about 75 seconds.

You can make up some whip cream in a mixing bowl while making the cake. Allow the cake to cool before you add the whipped cream on top!

Enjoy your dessert.

Chocolate and Peanut Butter Tarts

The last of the 15 keto recipes for weight loss the chocolate and peanut butter tart. Yes, this is another dessert, and it's definitely worth trying at least once. You'll want so much more of it!

You may question some of the ingredients. Avocado in a dessert? Well, this does work. Avocados tend to be bland on their own, so really soak in the flavors that you mix in.

Ingredients for the Crust:

¼ cup flaxseed ground until fine

2 tbsp almond flour

1 egg white

1 tbsp sweetener

Ingredients for the middle layer:

4 tbsp peanut butter (or nut butter of your choice)

2 tbsp butter

Ingredients for the top layer:

1 avocado

4 tbsp cocoa powder, unsweetened

¼ cup sweetener

½ tsp vanilla extract

2 tbsp double cream

½ cinnamon

Instructions:

1. Preheat the oven to 350°.

2. Mix the ground flaxseeds and rest of the crust ingredients until fully combined.

3. Press the mixture into a tart pan all the way up the sides.

4. Bake for 8 minutes until set.

5. Combine all the top layer ingredients in the blender. Smooth until creamy, and set to one side.

6. Allow the crust to cool, while mixing your peanut butter and butter in the microwave.

7. Pour into the crust and refrigerate for 30 minutes until set.

8. Now layer with your top layer. Smooth and place in the fridge for an hour or so.

Serve up this delicious dessert with some cream on the side. Your guests will love it, and will not notice the avocado.

Chapter 13

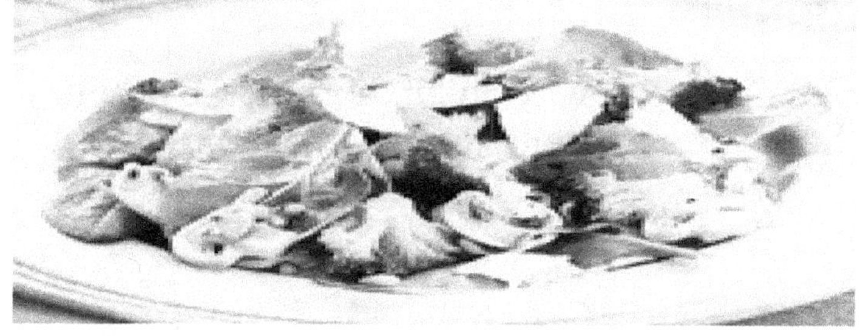

KETOGENIC DIET FOR VEGETARIANS

Is a ketogenic diet for vegetarians reasonably possible? Regardless of your motives for cutting out the animal meat, you are probably equally aware of all the buzz about the ketogenic diet, and wondering if you can go keto for all the performance while staying away from all the meats.

The answer is yes, but it takes a little extra thought. While the traditional keto diet typically involves a lot of meat for protein, it's also not necessary to eat meat while following the plan. In fact, the biggest component of the ketogenic diet is fat, which you can easily get from vegetarian foods.

For omnivores going keto, the most common mistake is eating too much protein.

However, the biggest mistake vegetarians make is eating too many carbohydrates from vegetables. You do have to be a little more careful with your carb and protein choices since traditional vegetarian forms of protein include things like beans and grains, which aren't a part of a keto diet.

Let's tackle this by discussing the three macronutrients one at a time.

CARBOHYDRATES FOR A VEGETARIAN KETOGENIC DIET

Since vegetarian diets are typically higher in carbs than meat-eating diets, it's especially important to understand the right types of carbs when following a meat-free ketogenic diet.

GOOD CARBS VS BAD CARBS

Besides getting plenty of healthy fats, watching your carbs is one of the most important factors here, and a lot of the go-to meals and especially snacks common for vegetarians and vegans are pretty carb-heavy. But excessive carbohydrates (even from veggies) aren't part of a keto diet. Of course, refined carbs like sugar, flour, bread, cereal, chips, etc. are immediately off the table.

BAD CARBS (HIGH GLYCEMIC, HIGHLY PROCESSED)

Here are some carb sources to remove from your home and kitchen:

Pastas

Breads

Chips, crackers, and pretzels

Tortillas

Rice

Sodas

Cereals

Any other packaged foods with refined sugars or flours.

Fruit juices and most fruits

White potatoes, sweet potatoes

Starchy vegetables

Good carbs on a vegetarian keto diet are basically the same as those on a normal keto diet, such as low-carb fruits, full-fat yogurts, and low-carb veggies.

GOOD CARBS (LIMITED) FOR A VEGETARIAN ON KETO

Low-carb Vegetables

If you're one of those vegetarians who hates vegetables, this diet is going to be harder for you. While the most important aspect of keto is keeping your fat content high, you'll need healthy low-carb veggies to provide enough bulk and fiber to fill in your meals and fill full at the same time.

Don't be afraid to explore and open yourself up to trying new vegetables in different ways. If raw turns you off, try cooking some in coconut oil or butter with lots of seasonings. Give yourself time to get used to the changes. Here are some low-carb vegetables to rely on:

Spinach

Kale

Collard greens

Swiss chard

Lettuce

Asparagus

Green beans

Broccoli

Cucumber

Summer and winter squash

Red and white cabbage

Cauliflower

Bell peppers

Onions

Mushrooms

Tomatoes

Eggplants

Garlic

 Fruits

All types of fruits should be limited, but berries are lower in sugars and carbs, so they're typically okay in small amounts, and at the end of the day before you fast while sleeping:

Blackberries

Strawberries

Raspberries

Blueberries

NON-CARBS TO MENTION (CONDIMENTS AND SPICES)

Condiments

If you can make all your condiments at home, that's the best choice, but these are okay to buy too. They are generally non-carbohydrate, or their carb count is microscopic.

Soy sauce or coconut aminos

Worcestershire sauce

Hot sauces

Yellow mustard

Mayonnaise (look for brands made with cage-free eggs)

Sugar-free ketchup

Sauerkraut (free of sugars)

Sugar-free or low-sugar high-fat salad dressings

Spices

Basil

Oregano

Parsley

Rosemary

Thyme

Cilantro

Cayenne pepper

Chili powder

Cumin

Cinnamon

Nutmeg

Lemon or lime juices

Pepper and salt

PROTEIN ON A VEGETARIAN KETOGENIC DIET

Here's a comprehensive list of protein-containing foods that have the green light on a keto vegetarian diet:

VEGETARIAN KETOGENIC PROTEINS

Eggs

Dairy

Tempeh

Natto

Miso

Nuts and seeds

If eating any soy products at all, try to stick to only those that are non-GMO and fermented (like organic tempeh).

If you find your protein needs still aren't being met, you could consider using an organic rice or hemp protein powder, but only use it as a supplement not a regular meal replacement. Also, just remember that getting too much protein is a common ketogenic diet mistake that prevents you from entering ketosis.

Be aware of packaged vegan and vegetarian meat substitutes: While these might be good substitutes for meat in terms of fat and protein, they might also contain a high amount of carbs. Be sure to check the carb content per serving, and consider the ingredients. Is it full or preservatives and fillers? Better meat substitutes would be any of the proteins mentioned above as well as portobello mushrooms or eggplant.

FATS FOR VEGETARIANS IN KETOSIS

NUTS AND SEEDS

Nuts and seeds are sources of both protein and fat. Just be sure to choose mostly low-carb and high-fat choices, as some nuts and seeds are higher in carbs than others, and can add up quickly.

Best nut options (lower carb):

Pecans

Brazil nuts

Macadamia nuts

Walnuts

Coconut (unsweetened)

Hazelnuts

Pine nuts

Almonds

Nut butters made from any of the above

Nut options to eat sparingly or not at all(higher carb):

Peanuts

Pistachios

Cashews

Chestnuts

Best seed options:

Chia seeds

Flaxseeds

HEALTHY OILS

The right types of oils are great for a ketogenic diet because they're entirely made of fat. MCT's in particular are a type of fat that is metabolized quicker than most, and broken down into useable energy. It also can easily cross the blood-brain barrier, which is why they are so beneficial to our mental clarity and performance.

Here are some more great options:

Olive oil

Coconut oil

Avocado oil

MCT oil

Macadamia oil

Flaxseed oil

Other Non-Dair Fat Sources

Olives

Avocados

Cocoa butter

Coconut cream

Dairy and Eggs

Heavy whipping cream

Cream cheese

Cottage cheese

Mayonnaise

Hard cheeses like parmesan, swiss, feta, and cheddar (full-fat)

Soft cheese like brie, Monterrey jack, mozzarella, and bleu cheese (full-fat)

Butter (grass-fed)

Eggs (make sure they're pastured or free-range and preferably omega-3-enriched)

Full-fat unsweetened Greek yogurt or coconut yogurt.

VEGETARIAN KETO MEAL IDEAS

Breakfasts

Vegetables and eggs with avocado fried in coconut or olive oil

Eggs frittata with asparagus and avocado

Vegetable and feta omelet fried in coconut or olive oil

Smoothie made from coconut cream, some berries, ice, full-fat yogurt, almond butter, and stevia extract

Lunch

Egg and avocado salad.

Mixed greens salad with avocado, mozzarella, pesto, olives, bell pepper, onions, a few nuts, lemon juice, and extra virgin olive oil dressing.

Vegetarian low-carb Greek salad with feta, tomatoes, onions, olives, fresh Greek spices, and extra virgin olive oil.

Stir-fried cauliflower "rice" with veggies and eggs.

Dinner

Cheese pizza with cauliflower crust and broccoli.

Pasta made with zucchini noodles and keto alfredo sauce.

Portobello "steak" with kale salad and cauliflower mashed potatoes.

Eggplant parmesan fried in coconut oil.

Okay, we are almost to the end of the post and I can hear you thinking...

What About Keto as a Vegan?

Great question. Since a vegan diet is even more restricted in terms of low-carb foods, keto as a vegan is highly impractical and takes a lot more thought. However, you can still consume plenty of fats if you stick to healthy oils, nuts/nut butters, avocados, seeds/seed butters, and coconut as your sources while making sure you get enough protein too.

Chapter 14

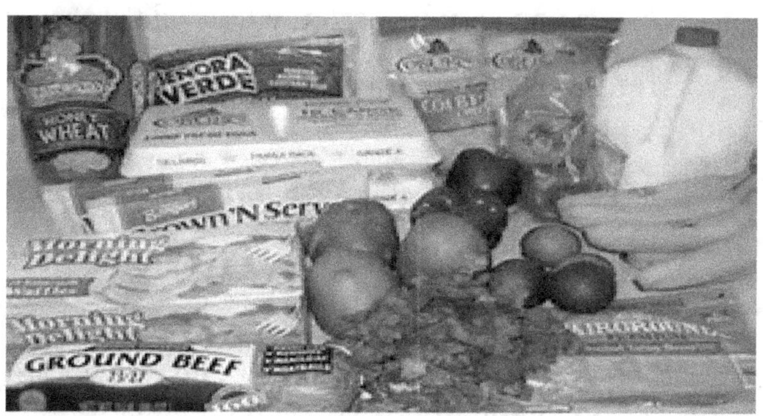

HOW TO DO THE KETOGENIC DIET ON A BUDGET

If your grocery budget is tight, but you still want to eat; well, don't worry. Eating a high-quality ketogenic diet on a budget is more than possible. It just takes a little extra planning, and staying clever with available resources. You may find you are saving money compared to quality high carbohydrate diets.

Many of us find that while we make some initial investment in overhauling our kitchen with ketogenic friendly foods and supplements, they end up saving money in the long-run. So not only is this chapter about how to do the ketogenic diet on a budget, it also shows how to examine if ketosis is actually helping your budget.

TIPS TO MAXIMIZE THE KETOGENIC DIET ON A BUDGET

BUY IN BULK

When you're trying to save money on food, bulk shopping is where it's at. It's tempting to shop at Whole Foods for

your items or even your regular local grocery store, but
you're not going to find bargain prices (most of the time)
this way, as much as you can; buy from wholesale stores.

And when you find a good deal there, take advantage!
Stock up, and plan to stretch it out. It's more money
upfront, but the savings can be ridiculous. Just make sure
you actually use the food you buy in bulk don't let it sit
forgotten in your freezer.

COOK IN BULK (AND FREEZE)

If you're already buying the food in bulk amounts cook in
bulk too! A lot of on-the-go foods you can buy just aren't
going to cut it when you're eating keto, so batch cooking
is an awesome way to make sure you always have meals
and snacks in the house. Not only will this save you
money, it'll save you time as well.

Choose one day each week to do your meal prepping and
cooking. Sunday works for most people, but it might be a
different day depending on your schedule. You might
choose to also do your shopping on the same day. The
day itself doesn't matter as long as you set aside time at
least once a week for each task.

Portion meals out into containers for easy grab-n-go. If
you're prepping for meals more than a week in advance,
you'll want to utilize that freezer space.

Enjoy your pre-portioned and prepped keto meals on a
budget without any extra work during the week. This way
will set you up for success.

LOOK FOR OFFERS & DISCOUNTS

Simple right? It only take a little bit of time to find some
awesome deals. When you shop at the grocery market,
look for deals and discounts, and be a hawk about it.

When meats are close to their expiration dates, stores will often discount them by as much as 20%. If you're cool with buying meat this close to expiration, this is a good opportunity to buy, and either use the food right away or freeze for later.

Pay attention to deals between the aisles too. Look for any "Buy 1, Get 1 Free" types of deals or discounts on foods.

You can really save a lot of money this way, so get used to keeping your eyes peeled for a good deal.

STICK TO A SHOPPING LIST

Without a clear list of what you're planning to buy, there's a 99.9% chance you'll end up buying more than you planned. Impulse buys are very real, and they get everyone. Having a list (and only buying what's on that list) is the best way to stick to your budget. This also gets easier as you get more familiar with your store, and know what types of deals you can expect each week. Oh yeah, and don't go shopping hungry.

USE A FOODSAVER

Along with freezing, get yourself a FoodSaver to vacuum seal your foods and make them last even longer. Plus, it'll make even more room in the freezer, which you'll need for bulk buying and cooking.

SHOP ONLINE

If you can't find the deals you want locally, or are short on time, shopping online is another viable option for saving that cash.

Check out Amazon for items like nuts, almond flour or coconut flour, coconut oil, flax or chia seeds, and spices. These are often cheaper to buy online than in the store, even with shipping.

Or, you can sign up for Amazon Prime to get that lovely free two-day shipping. They also offer free two-day shipping for six months to students; this is worth considering if you're still in school.   Another online resource is Nuts.com where you can buy nuts in bulk online at a discounted price.

STICK TO CHEAP VEGGIES

Buy vegetables that are a good deal, and that you can get a lot of use from. Broccoli and spinach are pretty good choices in most areas as far as cost goes, and they can be incorporated into just about any recipe. While cauliflower might not be the cheapest, it's so versatile (cauliflower rice or crust, etc) that it's worth the cost for most people.

DRINK CHEAP

Quit the pricey "diet" drinks and alcohol, and switch to water. It's what you should be drinking primarily anyway. If you need the caffeine, make your own coffee or tea at home in batches for the week, and carry them with you in a mug. No need to make that Starbucks run.

MAKE FOOD YOURSELF

Dressings, dips, flours, salsas, guacamole, nut butters, soups, salads... as much as possible, plan to make anything you could buy packaged yourself. Not only will it save you money, it'll eliminate a lot of added crap that shows up in processed foods at the store. You'll know exactly what you're putting in your body with homemade.

Keep these appliances front and center in your kitchen:

Food processor or blender

Pots and pans you don't need anything fancy, just some cookware that's high-quality enough to boil, fry, etc. each week

Knife and cutting board

Jars and containers for storing

This also goes for pre-chopped and frozen vegetables. Instead of spending more, take a little time to chop and store/freeze the veggies yourself.

Don't let budget concerns keep you from making your goals and your health a priority! Use what you have to make this diet work for you, even if it takes a little extra planning and preparing. Use these tips as a guide.

THE KETOGENIC BUDGET TIP – CALCULATE YOUR RETURN ON KETOSIS

In the grand scheme of things, what's is really more important than 50 cent coupons is long-term financial health, and long-term physical health.

Take the one-minute test and sketch a ledger to find your Return on Ketosis.

PART 1: QUANTIFIABLE RETURN ON KETO

Pull out a piece of scrap paper and answer these questions to the best of your ability. Don't spend too much time on it.

1. What are your meals like on keto vs. non-keto? Are you eating less volume and less frequently?

2. What are your beverages like? Are you consuming less alcohol and pre workout powder and caffeine?

3. What are your snacks like? Are you eating fewer snacks due to blood sugar spikes and crashes?

PART 2: GO DEEPER INTO QUALITATIVE RETURNS

Benefits of ketosis are:

Mental Performance

Clarity and focus

Physical Performance

Increased fat-burning

Boost energy for exercise

Increases satiety and feeling full

Psychological Performance

Sense of well-being

Emotional balance

Disease Prevention and Longevity

Ketosis induces improved autophagy and apoptosis, where your body purges dead or underperforming cells to allow for new growth. This has innumerable benefits relating to disease prevention, and longevity.

DOING KETO ON A BUDGET

A budget is a budget if you are in ketosis or not. Take these nine awesome practical tips to do the ketogenic diet on a budget, but then take a look at the wide-angle lens of your life and examine if ketosis is a worthy investment.

To expand on this topic, and even if keto is not right for you, is the price of being healthy worth it? Don't let budget concerns derail you. Many people in the first half of life waste their health trying to make money, and then in the second half of life they spend the money trying to get their health back.

Time to budget your time, energy, and hard-earned money into what really matters to you!

Conclusion

Thank you again for downloading this book!

Are you a meat lover, but need to lose weight? Then you might find yourself in a dilemma as most diets out there limit the intake of meat and other fatty food products because of high fat content, and calories as well. With that said, people who need to lose weight no longer have to be contented with eating carrot sticks or lettuce as one can now enjoy their favorite bacon and egg while still losing weight. The ketogenic diet, which once served as an epileptic prevention meal plan, is now being used by people who need to shed excess weight. There are 2 types the "long chain triglycerides" (LCT), and the medium chain triglycerides (MCT).

In a normal diet, humans need to consume higher amounts of carbohydrates as this acts as energy source for the body to be able to function well, and less of fat as fats are only stored in the body as a reserve for when the body needs more fuel. As the body needs more carbohydrates, it processes the food group after a while which is not so in the case of breaking down meals that are high in fat content.

Try to be mindful about the quality and quantity of foods you are consuming and staying away from processed foods. And at the end of the day, consult with your doctor, and possibly a nutritionist to find a plan that works best for your lifestyle.

Finally, if you enjoyed this book, then I'd like to ask you for a favor, would you be kind enough to leave a review for this book on Amazon? It'd be greatly appreciated!

Finally, if you enjoyed this book, then I'd like to ask you for a favor, would you be kind enough to leave a review for this book on Amazon? It'd be greatly appreciated!

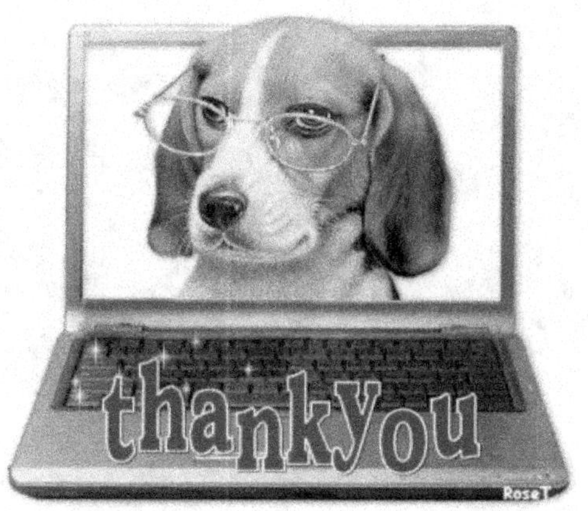

Thank you and good luck!

Preview Of 'GREEN THUMB PLANTING: HOW TO MAKE YOUR HOME GARDEN FLOURISH'

Chapter 1

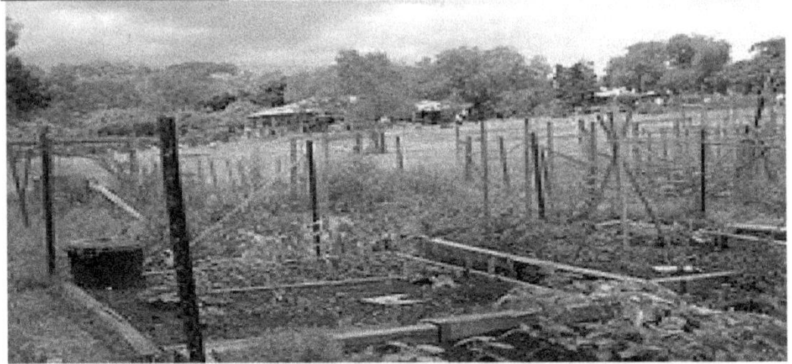

GREEN THUMB'S GUIDE TO A NEW GARDEN PLOT

When it comes to preparing a new garden plot, there are a lot of crucial factors a gardener must take into account that will shape the garden. You have to pick a suitable location, choose what sort of elements you're going to be putting in your soil, and how you're going to landscape your bit of earth. Here are a few tips to start off right for a beautiful, healthy garden.

The first step to preparing your plot is finding a good location. This is important when considering just what kind of garden you plan on growing, be it a flower garden, a vegetable plot etc. Do you need a shady area for plants such as ferns and fuchsia? Although most plants require lots of sunlight, some plants need partial shade, like snapdragons and columbines.

Are you growing leafy foliage that needs to be spread out over large amounts of space, or smaller plants that don't require much room? Consider what type of soil your garden needs: Dry sand or moist dirt? By figuring out what your plants need, you can decide the best location for your plot.

After you've selected the area for your plot, you're stuck with possibly the least enjoyable part of plotting a garden: clearing out all the unwanted vegetation that already lives there. Things like weeds and grass can ruin a garden before it's even finished. It is usually easier and generally more thorough to spray down a plot. However, many oppose weed killers and insecticides because they are said to be environmentally unsound. Thankfully, there are many organic substances that finish the job, and break down into nontoxic elements.

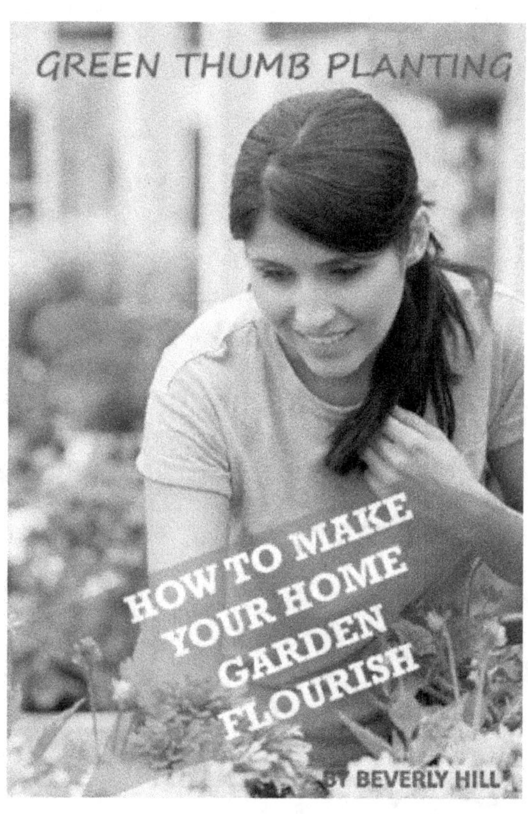

To check out the rest of (GREEN THUMB PLANTING: HOW TO MAKE YOUR HOME GAREDEN FLOURISH) go to Amazon.com

Check Out My Other Books

Below you'll find some of my other popular books that are popular on Amazon and Kindle as well. Alternatively, you can visit my author page on Amazon to see other work done by me.

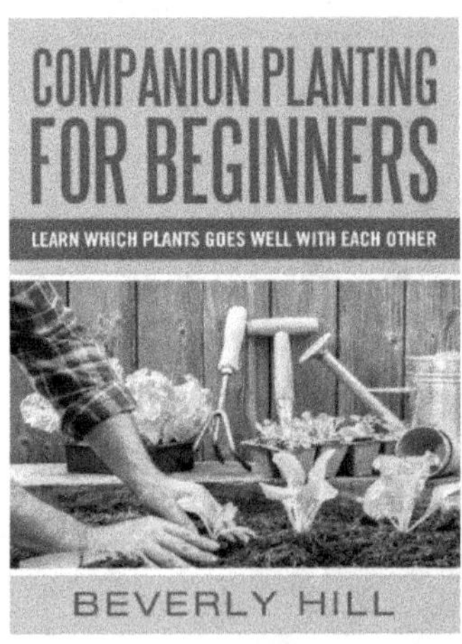

COMPANIOR PLANTING FOR BEGINNERS: LEARN WHICH PLANTS WORKS WILL WITH EACH OTHER.

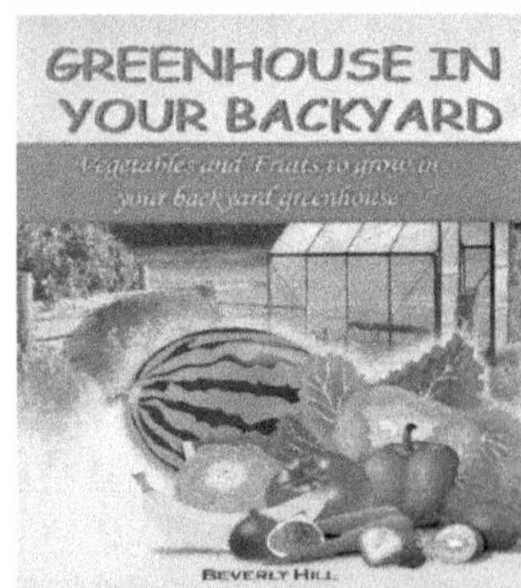

GREENHOUSE IN YOUR BACKYARD: VEGETABLES AND FRUITS TO GROW IN YOUR BACKYARD GREENHOUSE.

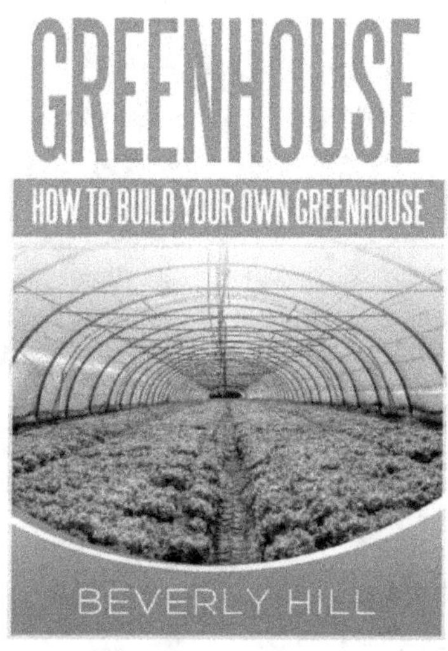

GREENHOUSE: HOW TO BUILD YOUR OWN GREENHOUSE.

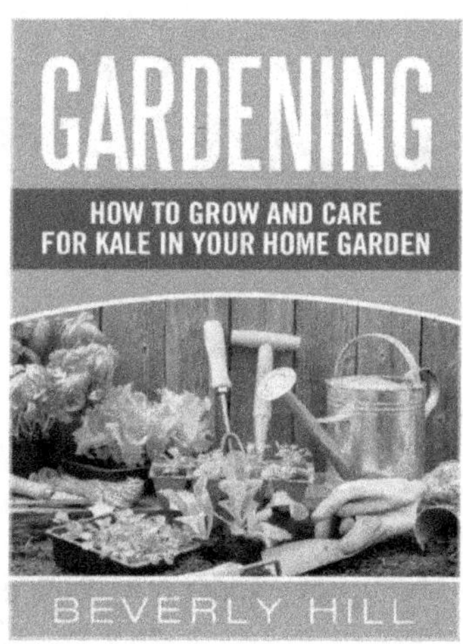

GARDENING: HOW TO GROW AND CARE FOR KALE IN YOUR HOME GARDEN.

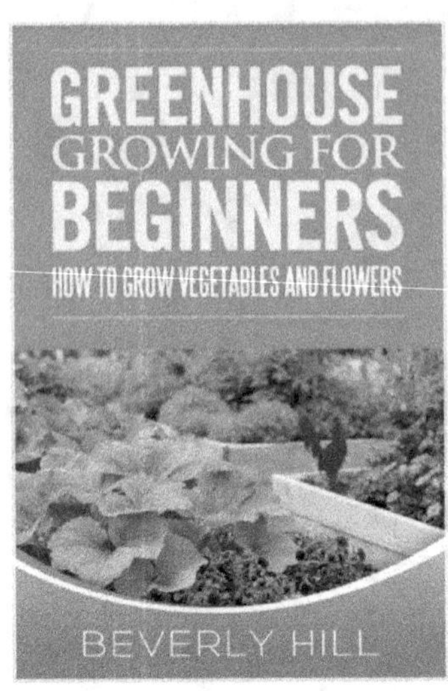

GREENHOUSE GROWING FOR BEGINNERS: HOW TO GROW VEGETABLES AND FLOWERS.

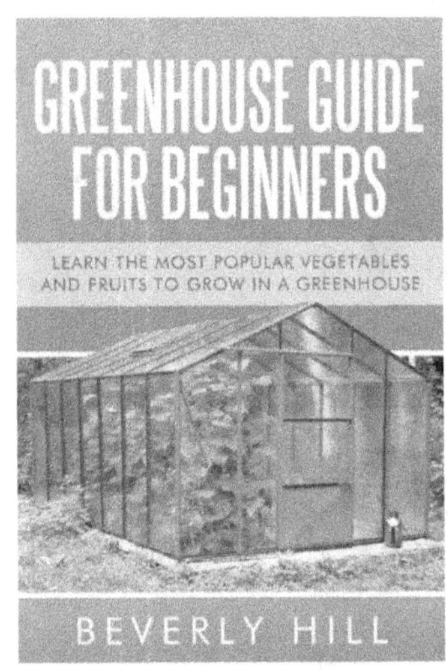

GREENHOUSE GUIDE FOR BEGINNERS: LEARN THE MOST POPULAR VEGETABLES AND FRUITS TO GROW IN A GREENHOUSE.

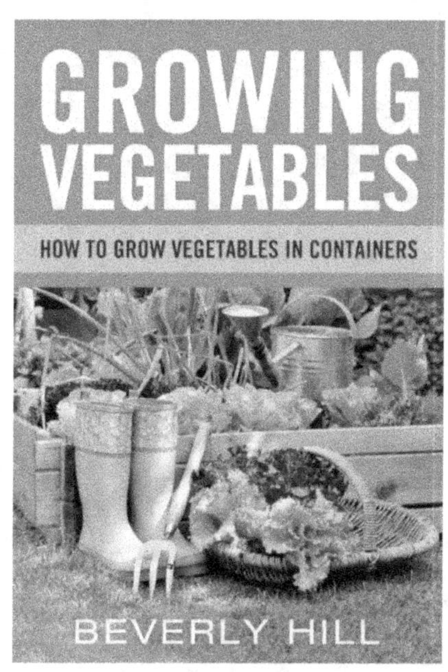

GROWING VEGETABLES: HOW TO GROW VEGETABLES IN CONTAINERS.

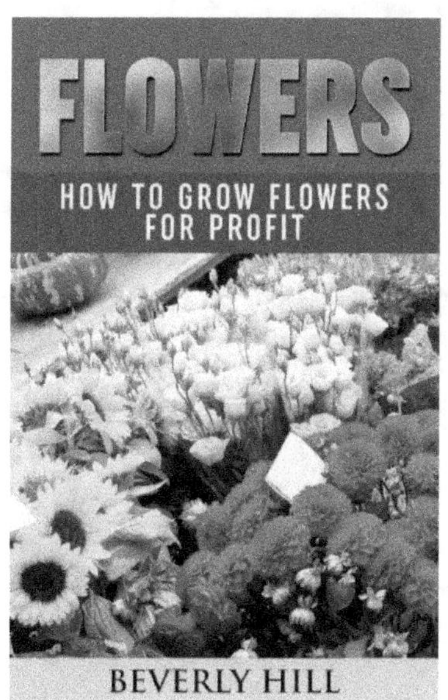

FLOWERS: HOW TO GROW FLOWERS FOR PROFIT.

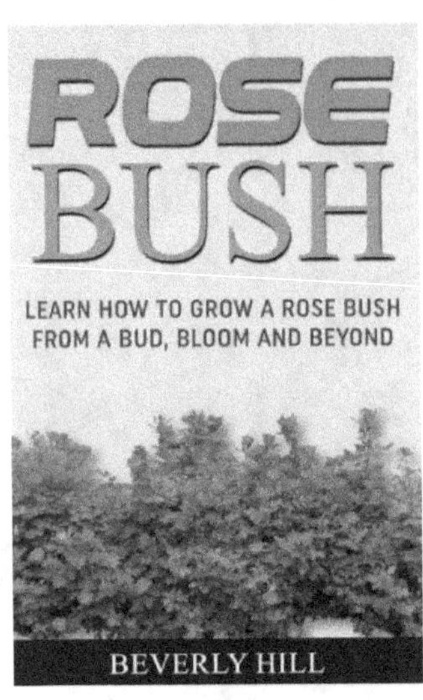

ROSE BUSH: LEARN HOW TO GROW A ROSE BUSH FROM A BUD, BLOOM AND BEYOND.

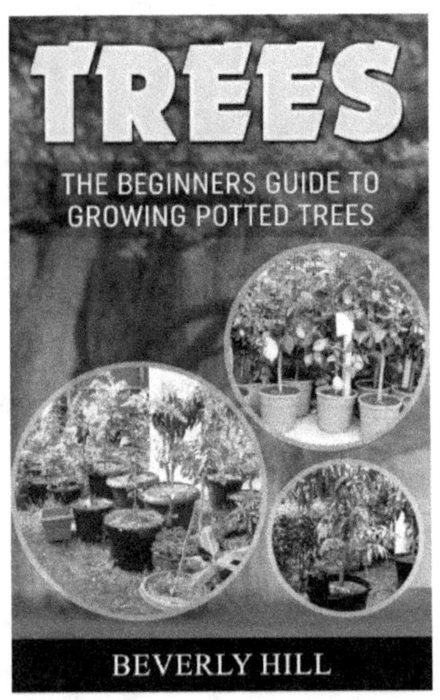

TREES: THE BEGINNERS GUIDE TO GROWING POTTED TREES.

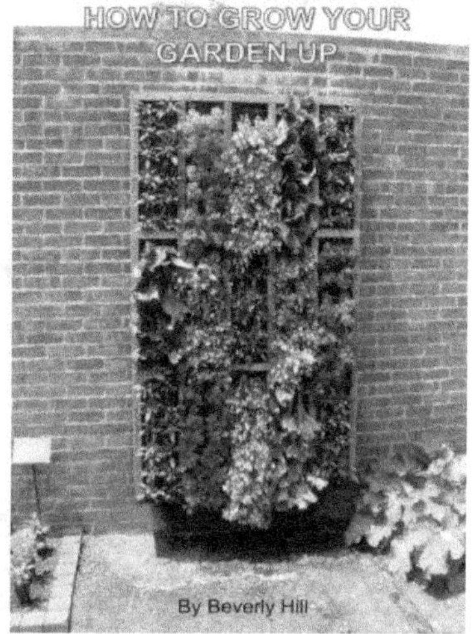

VERTICAL GARDENING: HOW TO GROW YOUR GARDEN UP.

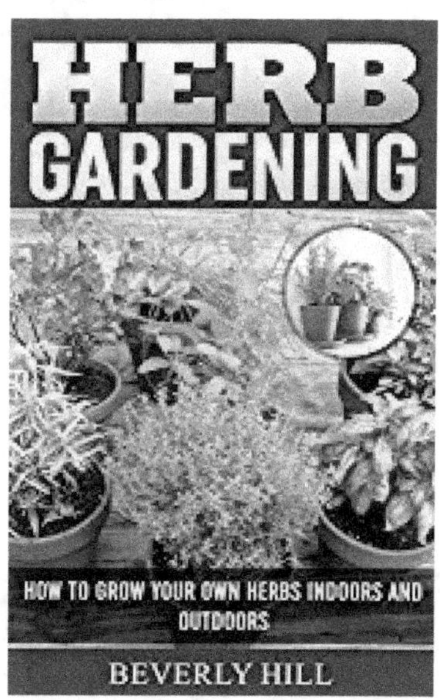

HERB GARDENING: HOW TO GROW YOUR OWN HERBES INDOORS AND OUTDOORS.

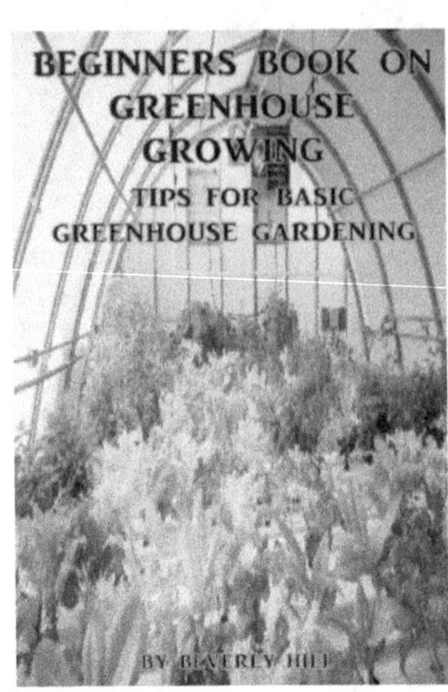

BEGINNERS BOOK ON GREENHOUSE GROWING: TIPS FOR BASIC GREENHOUSE GARDENING.

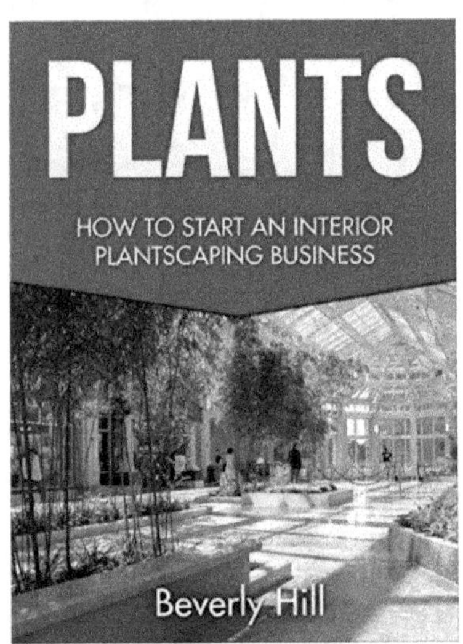

PLANTS: HOW TO START AN INTERIOR PLANTSCAPING BUSINESS.

BONUS: SUBSCRIBE TO THE FREE BOOK

Beginners Guide to Yoga & Meditation

"Stressed out? Do You Feel Like The World Is Crashing Down Around You? Want To Take A Vacation That Will Relax Your Mind, Body And Spirit? Well this Easy To Read Step By Step

E-Book Makes It All Possible!"

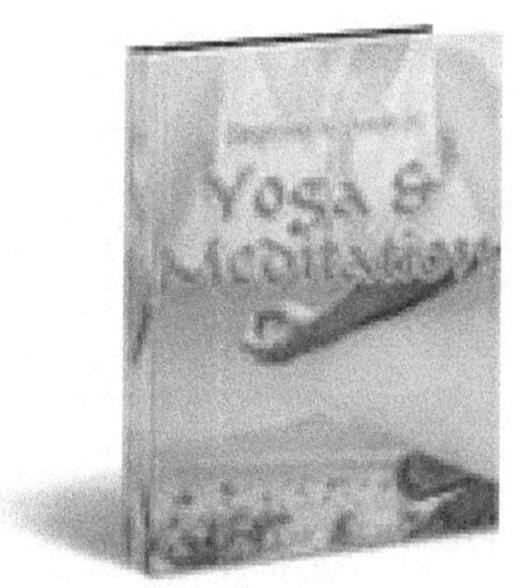

Instructions on how to join our mailing list, and receive a free copy of "Yoga and Meditation" can be found in any of my Kindle eBooks.

NOTES

NOTES

NOTES

* 9 7 8 1 9 7 4 6 7 1 9 7 7 *